THE HARVARD UNIVERSITY PRESS FAMILY HEALTH GUIDES

Chronic Pain and the Family

A NEW GUIDE

Julie K. Silver, M.D.

HARVARD UNIVERSITY PRESS
Cambridge, Massachusetts
London, England
2004

Library of Congress Cataloging-in-Publication Data

Silver, J. K. (Julie K.), 1965–
    Chronic pain and the family : a new guide / Julie K. Silver.
    p. cm. — (The Harvard University Press family health guides)
    Includes bibliographical references and index.
    ISBN 0-674-01505-3 (alk. paper; cloth) — ISBN 0-674-01666-1 (paper)
    1. Chronic pain—Patients—Family relationships—Popular works.
    I. Title. II. Series.
RB127.S499 2004
616'.0472—dc22
2004047527

This book is dedicated to my mentors, an eclectic group of very special people who have guided and inspired me both personally and professionally. I am blessed by and grateful for their presence in my life:

Dorothy Arnold
Diana Barrett
Walter Frontera
Lauro Halstead
Marc Shell

Contents

1   What Is Chronic Pain?   *1*

2   Effect on the Couple   *20*

3   Intimacy and Sexual Activity   *35*

4   Work Issues   *45*

5   Childbearing and Inheritance   *57*

6   Growing Up with a Parent in Pain   *64*

7   Chronic Pain in Children   *75*

8   The Extended Family   *86*

9   Emotional Changes and Depression   *95*

10   Medication Dependence and Addiction   *104*

11   Diagnosing Chronic Pain Conditions   *118*

12   Traditional Treatment Options   *124*

13   Complementary and Alternative Medicine   *139*

    Afterword   *148*

    Appendix: Resources   *151*

    Suggested Reading   *155*

    Notes   *159*

    Acknowledgments   *161*

    Index   *163*

CHRONIC PAIN AND THE FAMILY

1

What Is Chronic Pain?

Pain is an inevitable part of the human experience. We are born frail and vulnerable, and maturation does little to change our condition. Regardless of age, we have practically no natural protection from attacks by predators or even from the environment in harsh weather conditions. What keeps us safe is our intelligence and the ability to come up with methods to protect our soft skin, easily broken bones, and vulnerable vital organs. In fact, we humans live in mortal fear of even the slightest wound, and we have devised elaborate mechanisms to protect ourselves. Ironically, our intelligence is also the reason we suffer; our highly evolved brains are able to process and interpret pain. Most living species don't experience pain at all, or at least not in the manner that we humans do. So we pay a price for our keen intellect—we know firsthand what it means to suffer physical pain.

Although we all know what it's like to feel pain, the experience means something different to each of us. Thus deriving a definition for pain, an intangible experience that differs from person to person, can be challenging. Among medical practitioners pain is defined as an "unpleasant sensory and emotional experience associated with actual or potential tissue damage."[1] Despite this rather simple definition, most of us describe pain in other ways. We may describe pain by its characteristics (for example, sharp, burning, aching) or by its stimulus (hot, pricking, sharp). We can talk about pain's intensity (mild, moderate, severe) or use words to describe how we view it (miserable, annoying, intolerable). Despite the countless number of terms we can use to describe pain, however, there are only two things we can know for sure about someone else's pain: it's unpleasant and it's theirs alone to experience physically.

But just because others can't actually feel our pain doesn't mean they aren't affected by it. Family members are significantly impacted when one member is ill. When someone is *chronically* ill, as is the case with a chronic pain condition, the family is often thrown into turmoil. Defining how a family functions "normally" when everyone is healthy is nearly as impossible as defining "normal" family functioning when someone becomes ill. After all, what is "normal" when someone's world has been irrevocably altered? How do people function normally when they are plagued with pain, unable to work in their usual manner or maintain intimate relationships with their spouses? Similarly, what is normal for an "unaffected" family member such as a child who, when a parent becomes ill, must suddenly be quiet in the house or take on extra responsibilities and chores because the parent is unable to do them? Pain, in fact, is the quintessential solitary experience only in that the person affected is the only one who can *physically feel the pain*. In all other respects pain—particularly chronic pain—is a familial experience that dramatically changes the dynamics of the family as a unit and the functioning of the individual members. This book addresses the impact of chronic pain on the sufferer as well as on his or her family, and suggests ways to help everyone cope with the new reality.

The History of Pain

Humans have been documenting their pain since ancient times. We have found evidence of suffering etched on Babylonian clay tablets, Persian leathern documents, and parchment scrolls from Troy. Chinese acupuncture originated back in 2500 B.C. to alleviate pain, and we still use it today. More recently, archaeologists have found interesting correlations between afflictions of the past and those of the present. For example, Dr. Juliet Rogers studied 3,000 skeletons from a graveyard in Barton-on-Humber, a small village in north Lincolnshire, England. The bones she studied were from the period 900–1850. Dr. Rogers found evidence of a number of arthritic conditions including osteoarthritis, psoriatic arthritis, and Reiter's and Paget's diseases. What she did not find was evidence of rheumatoid arthritis. This led to the hypothesis that perhaps rheumatoid arthritis is a fairly "new" disease or at least one that is more common now than it once was. In this way the past may help us understand illnesses we encounter now, though many questions will likely remain unanswered. What is clear is that pain has been a consistent theme throughout human history.

Ancient peoples had many different belief systems to explain pain and illness in general. For example, in 8000 B.C. healers used very sharp instruments to cut holes in the skulls of people while they were still alive—a procedure now known as trepanning. We don't know for sure why this was done, but one theory is that these holes let out the "bad demons" that caused illness. Similarly, Ancient Egyptians believed that gods or spirits of the dead caused illnesses. In ancient China, people believed in two opposing unifying forces, the Yin (feminine, negative, passive) and the Yang (masculine, positive, active). Sickness occurred when these forces were out of sync with each other. Physicians were often religious men whose treatment centered on their theological beliefs and could include prayers, exorcisms, and incantations, among other things.

As the understanding of pain evolved, modern societies began to focus on the physical diagnosis of the underlying problem and then treatment, if available, for that condition. Yet despite many advances in pain medicine, there is currently no one theory to explain why pain occurs. This can be frustrating not only for the person who is suffering but for the entire family, all of whom want "answers" when they go to the doctor. Although we have come a long way since army surgeons in the 1500s treated what they thought were poisonous gunshot wounds by pouring burning oil over them, there is still much we don't know about pain and healing. It is beyond the scope of this book to discuss the current debates in pain medicine. Rather, I will focus on how pain, when it persists and becomes chronic, affects the person who is ill and his or her loved ones.

If you are living with chronic pain, it's important for you to understand how your condition and your reactions to it affect the people you love. If you are the loved one of someone who is suffering chronic pain, you need to know how best to respond to a situation that can often transform the entire family. Reading this book is a great place to begin. Obviously, you can't absorb or take over someone else's pain, but you can certainly *imagine* what pain must be like for your loved one. Great writers and artists through the ages have depicted pain with pictures and words to allow us to experience vicariously the pain of others. For example, in the *Iliad*,

Homer describes with grim detachment the gory details of brutal combat. We know from historians that Napoleon's men would continue to fight with amputated limbs, and artists have drawn great battle scenes depicting this phenomenon. Understanding chronic pain in your own family begins with empathy for the person suffering, but also involves encouraging yourself or your loved one to live as full and active a life as possible *despite the pain.*

The Language of Pain

Descriptions of others' pain can elicit great empathy from us. The novelist Fanny Burney left a detailed account of the mastectomy she underwent without anesthesia on September 30, 1811 (ether had not yet been invented). With only a wine cordial (perhaps with laudanum) to calm her, she watched through a transparent handkerchief draped over her face as the surgeon marked the spot on her breast where he would plunge his knife. Burney writes of the knife "cutting through veins—arteries—flesh—nerves" as the surgeon began "cutting against the grain." She describes her agonized screams as he scraped at her breastbone—screams that lasted throughout the surgery. Burney writes of her primal response, "I almost marvel that it rings not in my Ears still . . . so excruciating was the agony."[2]

Pain has its own language. Burney's screams resonate with us, even though her surgery was approximately two centuries ago. We know how pain is expressed—grunts, roars, groans, moans, sobs, cries, screams, and shrieks. When someone we love is in pain, we want to do whatever we can to help. When we are in pain, we want to be helped, to be relieved of the "unpleasant sensory and emotional experience associated with actual or potential tissue damage." To be relieved of pain. But even more than that, we want to be relieved of *suffering.*

In the case of chronic pain, however, language can become a problem. In the pain literature, the language of pain is often referred to as "pain behaviors." In general, pain behaviors are things that people do or say to let others around them know they are suffering. Often these behaviors stem from a need to inform others that the pain is real and the suffering genuine. Pain behaviors can manifest in many ways and may include constant or intermittent moaning, groaning, rubbing the neck or back, grimacing, limping, or constantly changing positions. People who are in pain often fall into a pattern of continually calling attention to their suffering, to no real advantage and often to their own detriment. For example, a person who moans frequently in response to pain does not change the physical experience. But the moaning may cause a spouse to respond in either an overly solicitous manner or with hostility and resentment.

Both responses tend to have negative effects on the person in pain and on the relationship in general. The overly solicitous spouse who constantly responds in a supportive and loving way to pain behaviors reinforces the disability of the person in pain and can even encourage more pain behaviors and less physical activity—all without a real change in the physical condition. At the other extreme, when a spouse becomes frustrated, resentful, or even outwardly angry, the effect on the person in pain and other family members who witness this breakdown in the relationship can be disastrous.

Pain behaviors are widely regarded as "maladaptive," meaning they serve no real purpose and can be very detrimental. It's critical for people in pain and their family members to recognize these behaviors and to work to change them. Effective communication comes not in the persistent moaning of someone in pain but rather in honest and loving communication.

The literature supports both a cultural and a gender role in the language and experience of pain. For example, it is well known that many more women than men seek out and receive treatment for pain. Women typically report more pain (especially musculoskeletal), a higher severity of pain, and pain for a longer duration of time. We don't know definitively why women are more likely than men to seek help. This phenomenon may be due to psychosocial factors such as society's willingness to tolerate "sensitive" women who express themselves and give voice to what is bothering them, and powerful social taboos against men expressing pain. Biological factors such as sex hormones and the different musculoskeletal structure of women may also play a role.

Cultural and socioeconomic differences may also be factors in how people respond to pain. For instance, some studies have indicated that certain cultural groups may be less inhibited than others about expressing their pain. Socioeconomic influences go hand in hand with cultural differences. For example, people from poor economic backgrounds may

How to Eliminate Chronic Pain Behaviors

PERSON IN PAIN

- Use words to describe what you're experiencing. Keep in mind, though, that people don't constantly need to hear exactly how you're feeling. There are many times when "suffering in silence" will be beneficial to you and your family members.

- Don't hold your spouse or other loved ones responsible for your physical comfort. If you need something and can get it yourself, then do so.

- Try to avoid canceling plans with people—it's disappointing for them and for you. If you can manage the activity, then go ahead and do it.

- Understand that the less active you are, the more pain you'll have as a result of physical deconditioning. So try to remain as active as possible.

- If you're unable to handle household responsibilities that were once yours, then take on new ones that you can manage in order to lessen the burden on your loved ones.

- Be your own advocate and seek legitimate medical treatment. Follow your doctor's advice unless there is a compelling reason not to. If you don't want to do something your doctor recommends, then discuss this with him so that an alternate treatment plan can be implemented.

- Engage in regular, but not incessant, honest and open communication with your family members about what's happening to you and how you're feeling. Ask them how they're feeling and listen with empathy. Remember that just because you're feeling the physical pain doesn't mean they're not suffering as well.

FAMILY MEMBERS

- Don't constantly ask how your loved one is feeling—particularly when the person is not complaining or focusing on the pain.

- Encourage the person in pain to do whatever he can to help himself and the family.

- Avoid taking over all the responsibilities for the family—ask and expect the pain person to help whenever possible.

- Don't be the go-between for the pain person and the doctor—they should have their own relationship, and the person in pain should be responsible for following through with all treatment plans.
- Don't cancel your plans to do things just because someone else is in pain. Enjoy the things that you can do. Keep in mind that children often cope the same way their parents do. If your children see you shut down and become reclusive, they may do the same. On the other hand, if they see you enjoying yourself and having fun despite difficulties at home, they will likely respond in kind.
- Engage in honest and loving communication on a regular basis with both the person in pain and other members of the family who may be affected as well.
- Don't respond to maladaptive pain behaviors. If you can, point out these behaviors in a loving way and try to reinforce the fact that they're not useful.

view pain as a tremendous threat to their employment and even to their survival. In societies where anesthesia is not routine for dental procedures, either because it is not available or because it is not customary to use it, children and adults often undergo what many people would regard as agonizing surgery without complaint. As with the gender disparity, cultural and socioeconomic differences clearly affect the language and experience of pain, though we don't know exactly why.

Virtuous Pain

None of us wants to experience pain or, worse yet, live daily with unrelenting pain. But is pain intrinsically bad? Is there anything redeemable about something that causes so much suffering? Obviously there are times when pain is useful. For instance, the very uncomfortable burning pain we feel when we touch a hot pan tells us to remove our hand immediately or we will suffer further injury. It's not uncommon for individuals with paraplegia and loss of sensation in their legs to inadvertently injure themselves by spilling hot coffee or some other substance without being aware that they had done so. Just about every doctor has a story about a patient with diabetic neuropathy (a condition that causes loss of sensation primarily in the feet) who walked around barefoot and stepped on a sharp object without even realizing it.

In his book *The Culture of Pain,* David Morris describes a man named Edward H. Gibson, a vaudeville stage act billed as the Human Pincushion.[3] Gibson would walk on stage and allow audience members to stick pins in him anywhere except the groin and the abdomen. During one show, Gibson thought he would do a reenactment of the Crucifixion. A woman in the audience immediately fainted when a man with a sledgehammer drove the first spike into Gibson's left hand. As Morris notes, Gibson wisely canceled the show. An audience that could tolerate watching a man being pricked by small pins was not prepared to watch him mutilate himself—even if he didn't feel it.

Gibson most likely had what is known as a congenital insensitivity to pain. Children with this condition may die prematurely because they are more likely both to sustain serious injuries and to ignore the injuries when they occur. This condition has led to the belief that pain has great survival value for us. Every time we shift our legs because we ache from being in the same position or don't touch something that's hot, our bodies remind us that pain is a very useful sensation that helps us protect ourselves.

Understanding and Classifying Pain

One way doctors classify pain is by how long it has been present. This is clearly an artificial and arbitrary classification, but it helps guide appropriate treatment. Pain is classified temporally as either *acute* or *chronic.* Although acute pain is always pain that has been present for a short period of time and chronic pain is always pain that has been present for a long period of time, there is no agreement in the medical literature about *how* long pain needs to be present to be considered chronic. The most common minimum duration for a diagnosis of chronic pain seems to be six months. However, a better, but somewhat more subjective, definition of chronic pain is pain that persists after the expected time it takes for tissues to heal from a particular injury or illness. This means that acute pain is the pain we experience during the time when the tissues are newly injured or haven't completely healed.

Acute Pain

Acute pain typically occurs with an injury, illness, surgery, or childbirth and is generally triggered by tissue damage. An example of acute pain that we have all experienced is a scratch. Although a scratch is certainly not a serious injury, it's a good example of how our bodies react to tissue damage. At the moment a scratch occurs, sensory nerve impulses travel from the skin to the spinal cord and brain, initiating not only the painful response we feel but also our bodies' first-aid response, which will allow the scratch to heal. Most of us don't live in fear of getting a scratch—we know that scratches are impossible to avoid, result in minimal pain, and heal quickly.

It's interesting to note that even with a much more serious injury such as the traumatic amputation of a finger, a knife or bullet wound, or a severely broken bone, the injured person often doesn't experience pain right away. Numerous reports have documented the experiences of soldiers in battle who, despite gaping wounds, cannot recall feeling pain until long after they were injured. Other studies have examined people who arrive in emergency rooms with fresh wounds but report a pain-free period after being injured. It's not clear why some people don't experience pain immediately after a very traumatic injury, as would be expected. It may be that they're exhilarated because they're just wounded and not dead; it may be that they're in shock; or it may be that they're so focused on getting medical treatment that they simply don't feel the pain. Certainly the sympathetic nervous system, which kicks into high gear during times of extreme stress and releases a variety of chemicals in what is called a "fight or flight" response, plays a role in this phenomenon.

Surgery is another example of severe acute pain that results from extensive tissue damage. In his book *Pain: The Science of Suffering*, Patrick Wall, a professor of physiology and an authority on pain, writes, "Entry into the hospital involves a rite of passage to translate the person from free citizen to dependent patient. Forms are filled out with an implicit threat. Next of kin and religion are requested. A permission form is signed that transfers responsibility to others. The patient is stripped of familiar clothes and dressed in a silly gown in a strange room with strange people."[4] After the surgery most people have pain, but the severity can vary widely. For the post-operative patient whose pain is not controlled, and whose nurse may not be empathic (and very often is waiting for a busy surgeon's pain medication orders), the ordeal of surgery, regardless of whether it accomplished the goal of fixing a hernia, taking out a tumor, or delivering a baby, is a disaster.

Healthcare providers sometimes forget what a difficult and potentially humiliating experience having surgery can be. But it used to be much worse. In the days before ether, the first general anesthesia, people underwent surgery much as Burney described her mastectomy. The options were limited: alcohol, laudanum, and physical restraint were the main methods available to "help" someone through surgery. Hypnosis was also commonly used.

It's no secret that treating patients' pain adequately has not always been a priority in the hospital setting. The medical community is beginning to recognize the importance of treating acute pain, so much so that pain is now considered the "fifth" vital sign, after temperature, pulse, respiratory rate, and blood pressure. When hospitals undergo accreditation, they must show documentation that during admission patients' vital signs are taken and they are asked whether they are in pain. According to the *Comprehensive Accreditation Manual for Hospitals: The Official Handbook,* "The following statement on pain management is posted in all patient care areas (patient rooms, clinic rooms, waiting rooms, etc.) . . . *All patients have a right to pain relief.*"[5] Medical personnel are now required to show that they work together with patients and families to "establish a goal for pain relief and develop and implement a plan to achieve that goal." These regulations are a very important step in trying to make pain relief a priority for every patient who enters the hospital.

We have all experienced acute pain ourselves and have helped others with acute pain. Whether the situation calls for bandaging a child's scratched knee or calling "911," we know how to respond to acute pain situations. In most cases, there is a period of intensity as we work to help ourselves or another person who is injured; this period is followed by relief and a return to "life as usual" when the acute pain is taken care of. Acute pain rarely affects family members for more than a brief period of time. Unless the injury is horrific, the crisis quickly resolves and there is no lasting impact on the individual or the family (though of course parents usually remember a child's suffering). With chronic pain there is no such resolution. Indeed, the impact of chronic pain on family members is lasting and transformative.

Chronic Pain

Eight out of ten outpatient visits to physicians are for conditions with a pain component. Although accurate statistics are not available, it is estimated that approximately 25–30 percent of Americans live with chronic pain, and that up to 50 percent of us will suffer from chronic pain at some time during our lives. Moreover, the older we get, the more likely we are to live with chronic pain. In fact, studies show that 80–85 percent of older adults have conditions in which pain is a prominent feature. Chronic pain is estimated to cost as much as 100 billion dollars annually in lost work productivity, lost revenue, and medical expenses. Not surprisingly, chronic pain is a leading cause of disability. Those who suffer from it are affected in every aspect of their lives. They may be unable to work, exercise, or participate in activities with their children. They may not be able to enjoy a satisfactory sex life with their spouses or share the daily responsibilities of childrearing and maintaining a household. Chronic pain can be devastating to the person experiencing the pain as well as to the entire family unit.

Unlike acute pain, chronic pain is not always related to actual tissue damage. In fact, chronic pain can be present long after all the injured tissues have healed. It's not clear what causes someone to continue to experience pain after the usual time of healing, but most likely it has to do with chemicals that are triggered in the brain.

Chronic pain can also occur in someone with an ongoing disease such as arthritis. When this is the case, there is no definitive period of acute pain during which the tissues heal. Rather, there is ongoing destruction of the cartilage that protects the joints and keeps the bones from rubbing against each other. As the arthritis progresses, so does the intensity and duration of the pain. This type of chronic pain is associated not with a healing process gone awry but rather with the progressive nature of a disease that cannot be arrested or cured.

Chronic pain may also present as pain that is not due to a particular injury but rather occurs insidiously over time without an obvious reason.

This is often the case with pain in the neck, low back, pelvis, and various other parts of the body. Studies done specifically on pelvic pain have demonstrated no identifiable cause for the symptoms in 75 percent of cases. Statistics for low back pain are similar. Muscle pain syndromes such as fibromyalgia or myofascial pain conditions are examples of this type of chronic pain as well. Consequently, when someone is experiencing chronic pain, he or she often has the additional burden of not being able to understand why the pain is continuing long after an acute injury has healed, or why, when there was no injury to begin with and there is no identifiable cause for the pain on testing, it exists at all. For people who have a known disease that is progressive and incurable, such as rheumatoid arthritis, understanding the reason for the pain may bring little solace.

Regardless of whether there is a known cause for the pain someone is experiencing, the pain alone is often not responsible for the suffering. Many people live with pain on a daily basis and see it as little more than an annoyance. So what happens when someone has pain and begins to *suffer*? The anguish really begins when someone's life is curtailed, when dreams go by the wayside, and when day-to-day activities become onerous or even impossible. Suffering occurs when relationships with family members are strained and sexual and emotional intimacy with one's spouse is affected. The entire family suffers when there's a loss of income because a parent or spouse can no longer work. So suffering is really a manifestation not of pain itself but of the losses that occur when pain persists. It is the loss of *function* that causes suffering. When someone in pain seeks treatment, the physician faces the *suffering* individual and not just the pain.

Often this loss of function is gradual. Since chronic pain generally waxes and wanes in intensity, people report having good days and bad days. On the good days, they often try to make up for lost time, doing extra chores, taking a long walk, or even making love. This increased activity may lead to intensifying pain and a few bad days in a row. During the bad days, it's hard to do much because the pain is severe. Then, when another good day comes, the person in pain may remain very sedentary out of fear of triggering more pain and more bad days. This cycle of increased pain with activity, particularly unaccustomed activity, followed by rest and the fear of becoming more active again leads to physical deconditioning and even more pain.

The change in lifestyle that often accompanies chronic pain is not confined to the person in pain. Medical bills pile up at the same time that there may be a loss of income. The entire family may be unable to maintain their standard of living. Even if finances are not an issue, day-to-day life for the entire family may change. A once-active parent who loved to take the family hiking and coached the children's sports teams may now be sedentary and unable to do those things. Couples may experience a role reversal when the primary breadwinner suddenly stops working or cuts down on hours. This new situation may shift the at-home responsibilities to the pain person, who may not be able to manage the chores, shopping, cooking, or yard work very effectively. Most families have plans for the future and these plans may no longer be realistic. The loss of long-held goals, dreams, and plans might make the family frustrated and even resentful.

Just as the family is affected when a loved one is in pain, so the person in pain is influenced by the family's response to the situation. Obviously, when a spouse or parent isn't doing all the things he or she used to do, the other members of the family will be affected. But what might not be so apparent is that the family's reactions to and understanding of the pain issues can significantly impact pain and suffering. For example, studies have shown that family perceptions can greatly influence the medical treatment someone receives. The concern that family members express about a loved one's becoming dependent on medications may result in a patient being under medicated. This is particularly true in cases such as terminal cancer, where high-dose opiates are the treatment of choice. Some family members may scoff at complementary or alternative medical options that could potentially benefit the person in pain. Spouses might try to talk their loved ones out of treatments such as corticosteroid (that is, cortisone) injections because they have heard from friends that these have unpleasant side effects (many people erroneously believe that injected corticosteroids will cause weight gain and other side effects). On the other hand, a well-meaning spouse may encourage her partner to seek medical treatment relentlessly in the hopes of finding a cure for the condition or the pain. The spouse may convey to the pain person that he is not trying hard enough, a situation that may result not only in unnecessary medical consultations but also in inappropriate medical treatment that could potentially worsen the condition. The fear of never being out of pain or of having to live the rest of one's life with someone who is in chronic pain can make people take desperate actions. For all these reasons it's important to be aware of the family's influence on someone who is living with chronic pain.

Common Painful Conditions

We all anticipate pain, knowing that it's unavoidable. For some people, though, the thought of having pain, or having *more* pain than they're currently experiencing, is terrifying. Pain can be an unwanted sign of aging to some people. To others, it may be an indication that their previous good health is a thing of the past. Fear of pain is also universal. In 1918 Enid Bagnold wrote, "Isn't the fear of pain next brother to pain itself?" But it's not pain alone that concerns many people. Rather, they fear their ability, or lack of ability, to handle the pain they experience with *dignity*. In this section I list some common painful conditions. This is not meant to be an all-inclusive list, nor is it meant to be discriminative and exclude any particular condition. It is simply a short compilation of common medical conditions that cause people considerable pain and suffering.

Arthritis

The most common type of arthritis is degenerative ("old-age") arthritis, usually called osteoarthritis. There are other, more progressive and disabling types of arthritis such as rheumatoid arthritis. In general, arthritis occurs when the cartilage that is used to cushion and protect the joints deteriorates. Most often this is a result of age and general wear and tear on the joints. Osteoarthritis occurs equally in men and women. Early symptoms of osteoarthritis include morning stiffness and sometimes pain. As the disease progresses, the pain can occur throughout the day and becomes more severe. Treatment for osteoarthritis depends on which joints are affected, how much pain and disability someone is suffering, and the severity of the loss of cartilage.

Back Pain

Back pain is something nearly all of us will experience at some point in our lives. Fortunately, for many people the pain is short-lived. However, millions of people will go on to suffer from chronic back pain—most commonly in the low back region. Although we have very sophisticated imaging studies such as MRI (magnetic resonance imaging) scans and CT (computed tomography) scans, much of the time it's impossible to locate the exact source of the pain. This is most likely because the pain occurs at a more microscopic level than what can be demonstrated by modern technology. Presumably most back pain is due to muscle strains and ligamentous sprains. In more serious cases, the nerves or the spinal cord may be involved. When the lower lumbar or sacral nerves are involved, people often call this "sciatica." Although the sciatic nerve is not usually the culprit, many people understand this term to mean that there is pain radiating from the back to the leg—often causing numbness and/or tingling. The real source of this pain is typically a nerve that's a little higher up than the sciatic nerve. Nerves in the back (and neck) can be compressed by a "herniated" disk or by bony structures that form the spinal column. Despite the fact that more often than not the exact source of back pain cannot be found, in general when there is pressure on a nerve it's usually much easier to determine the location of the problem. The prognosis for back pain depends not only on the etiology of the pain but also on its longevity, response to treatment, and other factors.

Face Pain

Face pain can be due to a variety of factors, including misalignment of the jaw and teeth or poor dental hygiene that leads to chronic cavities in the teeth and gum disease. Face pain can be quite severe and debilitating. It also can be highly treatable—depending on the underlying cause.

TEMPOROMANDIBULAR JOINT DISORDERS

Temporomandibular joint pain, or TMJ, as it is often called, is a term used to refer to pain that is located in the jaw and is not directly related to pathology in the teeth or gums. Studies reveal that up to 25–30 percent of people may experience some symptoms of TMJ, which is five times more common in women than in men. Typical symptoms, other than jaw pain, include noises such as popping, clicking, grinding, and crepitation (a crunching sound). Associated symptoms are headaches and neck pain. Treatment varies but can include medications, mouth guards, orthodontic work (for example, braces), injections, and surgery.

TRIGEMINAL NEURALGIA

Trigeminal neuralgia is also known as *tic douloureux*. This pain typically occurs on the side of the face and is frequently caused by a blood vessel pressing on the trigeminal nerve. This nerve is very sensitive and controls sensation in the face and some of the chewing muscles. This condition is most common in people between the ages of fifty and seventy, though it can occur in younger adults. Symptoms are usually intermittent but can be very severe and "shock-like." Treatment generally involves medication, though surgery is sometimes indicated.

Headaches

Headaches are the most common and familiar cause of pain. Nearly everyone has experienced a headache, and most people get headaches intermittently throughout their lives. Headache pain can run the gamut from virtually unnoticeable to crippling. Although there are many different kinds of headaches, the two most common types are tension and migraine.

TENSION-TYPE

Tension headaches account for approximately 90 percent of all headaches. They range from mild to severe and generally consist of a gradual dull or tight feeling that occurs on the forehead, scalp, back of the neck, or sides of the head. The pain may feel like pressure or sometimes burning or throbbing. Tension-type headaches appear to be due to the tightening of the muscles around the neck and head. Something that causes these muscles to go into spasm can thus trigger a headache. Common factors can include working for a long time at a computer, talking on the phone with your neck bent to one side, wearing a tight hairband, or even stress that is accompanied by increased muscle tension. These headaches can occur sporadically or become chronic if the inciting factors are not addressed.

MIGRAINE

Author Joan Didion describes her migraine headaches in this manner: "That no one dies of migraine seems, to someone deep into an attack, an ambiguous blessing." Migraines are notorious for being incredibly debilitating, with throbbing pain sometimes accompanied by nausea and vomiting. Loud noises or bright lights may worsen the pain. The exact cause of migraines is currently under debate. For many years it was believed that these headaches were primarily due to constriction of the blood vessels. More recently, chemicals in the brain have been implicated as causative factors as well. Muscle tension may also contribute to migraine pain. Other factors include hormone fluctuations (women have migraines more commonly than men and often around the time of menstruation), diet (alcohol, aged cheeses, chocolate, and caffeine have all been noted to trigger some migraine attacks), environment (bright lights, strong odors, or changes in the weather may be factors), lifestyle (stress can bring on migraines), and medications (some medications may actually promote headaches). The treatment for migraines has improved significantly over the past decade. As our understanding of the cause of migraines advances, even more promising new treatments will become available.

Muscle and Soft Tissue Pain Syndromes

FIBROMYALGIA

Fibromyalgia is a syndrome (or collection of symptoms) that occurs more often in women than in men. The hallmark of fibromyalgia is widespread pain of at least six months' duration. The cause of fibromyalgia is not known, but it typically affects the muscles (causing tender points) and causes pain without inflammation. Other symptoms can include difficulty with sleep, digestive problems, and chronic fatigue. Fibromyalgia is diagnosed after other causes of pain are excluded, because a specific test for the condition does not currently exist. Treatment for fibromyalgia can be very successful and is usually aimed at keeping people active through exercise and lifestyle modifications, and utilizing other interventions such as medications, injections, acupuncture, and so on.

MYOFASCIAL PAIN SYNDROME

Myofascial pain syndrome is similar to fibromyalgia in that it involves muscular pain and spasm (tender points) and is diagnosed by excluding other testable causes of pain. It differs from fybromyalgia in the following ways: (1) it is more localized to a specific body region; (2) it occurs equally in men and women; and (3) it is far less likely to have associated symptoms of fatigue, irritable bowel, and sleep problems. The etiology of the symptoms is not known, but as the name suggests (*myo* = muscle and *fascial* = fascia accompanying the muscles), the presumed problem lies within the muscular structures. The treatment for myofascial pain syndrome is similar to that for fibromyalgia and may include posture retraining, exercise, medications, injections, and acupuncture, among other things.

Neck Pain

Neck pain is very common in people of all ages. It's often due to poor posture (for example, long hours at the computer or sitting in meetings). Muscle strains, ligament sprains, arthritis in the upper spine, and numerous other factors can also cause neck pain. Treatment is based on the underlying cause of the pain.

Abdominal Pain

Chronic abdominal pain can be due to a variety of factors including inflammatory bowel diseases, poor diet, constipation, and diverticulitis, among other things. Abdominal pain can be associated with psychological distress in both children and adults. Irritable bowel syndrome is a common cause of abdominal pain; some evidence suggests that people with this condition may have bowels that react more strongly to diet, activity, or stress than people without the condition.

Pelvic Pain

Pelvic pain generally occurs in women and may afflict up to 20–30 percent of women at some point in their lives. There are many muscles and ligaments in the pelvis that are prone to injury. Additionally, the pelvis contains the bladder and portions of the bowel, as well as the uterus (endometriosis occurs when pieces of the uterine lining migrate outside the uterine cavity), which can all cause pain if affected. In some cases pelvic pain with no other obvious causes may have a psychological component linked to a history of sexual abuse.

Foot Pain

Foot pain can be particularly disabling because we must bear weight on our feet in order to walk. Foot pain can occur for a multitude of reasons but is increasingly common as we age. Foot deformities such as bunions can contribute to pain. A primary consideration in foot pain is proper footwear. Someone with foot pain might want to consider shoes that are extra deep and wide. Occasionally other modifications such as a steel shank or a rocker bottom sole can markedly reduce pain. Medications, injections, physical therapy, braces, and surgery are also treatment options—depending on the underlying condition.

We can all expect to have pain in our lifetimes. While none of us wants to have chronic pain, in fact many of us will. If you or a loved one is living with pain, this guide can help. As with any medical condition, the more you arm yourself with knowledge, the better equipped you are to deal with it. The physical aspect of pain is, of course, only part of the story. The person in pain must also consider how his or her condition affects family members and even friends and coworkers. Only then can all aspects of the chronic pain be treated effectively. It is my hope that this book will be a valuable resource for you and your loved ones. The more people you share it with, the greater the chance that those who are close to you will understand how pain affects not only the individual but also the entire family.

2

Effect on the Couple

Chronic pain affects the spousal or other committed long-term relationship perhaps more than any other. Spouses often spend more time with each other than with anyone else, and the profound feelings they have for each other contribute to the significant effect that illness has on their marriage.

As with all relationships, chronic pain impacts a marriage in many ways. Although every relationship is different, there are some important factors that all partners should consider when their significant other suffers from chronic pain. First, the effect on the relationship is usually directly proportional to the frequency and intensity of the pain as well as the degree of disability. Someone with occasional severe migraine headaches may function normally most of the time, and so the impact on the spousal relationship will probably be minimal. By contrast, for someone who suddenly sustains a severe back injury, say, and is thereafter in chronic pain and unable to work, the effect on the couple may be very significant. Second, no two couples will handle the situation in the same way; some will adjust well despite a severe and debilitating injury, whereas others will find it difficult to cope after a lesser injury.

Research has shown that patterns of behavior for both the spouse and the person in pain may positively or negatively impact the marriage and the family dynamics. Couples facing chronic pain must consider what expectations each spouse has for the relationship. They would also do well to tap into any previous experience they have had in dealing with chronic illness. All of these things will likely influence how couples respond to living with chronic pain as a component of their relationship.

Loss of the Original Relationship

For most people, the wedding vows are said during a time of good health, when the words "in sickness and in health" do not have ominous over- tones. As we age with our loved ones, however, we begin to realize that eventually we will have to face the "sickness" part of those vows. In fact, doctors in my specialty, physiatry (physical medicine and rehabilitation), are fond of saying that "being able-bodied is a temporary condition." So what happens if you're forced to live with chronic pain or you're a well spouse who is faced with a partner who has chronic pain?

One of my patients is a newly married young woman who was hit by a car while jogging. Since her accident she has suffered from chronic pain and fatigue. Although she was out of work for months, she has now re- turned to her job as a buyer for a large department store chain. She finds the daily work taxing and the travel impossible. By the time she gets home from the office she's ready for bed. She has been struggling with depres- sion resulting from the loss of her marriage as she knew it. When she married she had thought this time in her life would be filled with happy outings with her husband as well as a lot of shared intimacy. Instead, she comes home exhausted, barely speaks to her husband, and sleeps for at least twelve hours each night. Her husband is unhappy because he is saddled with most of the chores; at the same time he feels as though he has lost his best friend. He rarely sees his wife between working and sleeping, and their sex life has suffered. Although they had planned to start a family soon, they have decided to wait because of the accident.

Most newlyweds enter marriage with certain expectations. We antici- pate defined roles. This doesn't mean that one person always does the cooking or that only one person is gainfully employed; it just means that there's typically agreement about how the daily responsibilities of mar- ried life will be handled. Although these roles may change over time, in marriages in which illness is not a factor, the roles change because the couple agrees to restructure the marital and family tasks. When one per- son becomes ill, however, the roles may change suddenly or gradually change over time without the consent or sometimes even the recognition of either partner. This can be devastating for both the well spouse and the person in pain. In general, the more disabled one partner becomes, the

greater the impact on the family and in particular the spousal relationship. This is why treatment for chronic pain is so *function*-oriented (during my medical training, the physiatrists who taught the residents would
routinely remind us to "focus on function"). The reasoning behind such
an approach is that if someone continues to function well, despite having
pain, his or her life will be much more fulfilling.

In 1960 the Holmes-Rahe Social Readjustment Scale was developed by
physicians Thomas Holmes and Richard Rahe to describe the disruptive
and stressful events that can occur in someone's life.[1] Despite the fact
that this scale was first introduced half a century ago, it continues to
be useful. I have modified the scale considerably to reflect what might
happen in a family where one person has chronic pain. The scale is perti-
nent to chronic pain because it's easy to visualize the enormous stress
that a couple (and family) might encounter when someone is chronically ill. Of the forty-three life events that may cause considerable stress,
thirty-four may happen as a direct result of chronic pain. The relevance
of some of these events to chronic pain might not be immediately obvious. For instance, we might wonder how a minor violation of the law
could be connected to chronic pain. When I asked one of the psychologists I work with whether she would include this category, however, she
said that she often sees people with chronic pain who have become so
frustrated that they run into trouble with the law. Common infractions
can include a traffic violation, public disturbance, or domestic violence.
Simply put, if you or your partner experiences chronic pain, you are particularly vulnerable to experiencing 75 percent of the most common and
stressful life events. Given this reality, it's easy to recognize the enormous impact that this condition can have on your marriage and your
family.

Maggie Strong is one of the first people to give voice to well spouses in
her book *Mainstay*. Strong lives with a husband who is chronically ill, and
she has become an advocate for well spouses (she's the founder of the
Well Spouse Foundation). Strong documents the enormous impact that
a chronic illness of any kind has on the healthy spouse. She describes
what she and her husband expected from their marriage: "we wanted a
marriage in which we both felt like equal partners. We'd each paid hom-
age to an older sibling and neither of us ever wanted to feel like the
smaller or weaker part of a twosome again."[2] According to Strong, the

Major Stressors

RANK	EVENT
1	Death of spouse
2	**Divorce**
3	**Marital separation**
4	Jail term
5	Death of a close family member
6	**Personal injury or illness**
7	Entering a new marriage
8	**Loss of job**
9	Marital reconciliation
10	**Retirement**
11	**Change in the health of a family member**
12	Pregnancy
13	**Problems with intimacy and sex**
14	Gaining a new family member
15	**Business readjustment**
16	**Change in financial state**
17	Death of a close friend
18	**Change to another line of work**
19	**Increased arguments with spouse**
20	**Difficulty paying household bills**
21	**Foreclosure of a mortgage or loan**
22	**Change in responsibilities at work**
23	Son or daughter leaving home
24	**Trouble with in-laws**
25	**Lack of outstanding personal achievement**
26	**Spouse beginning or stopping work**
27	**Going back to school or retraining**
28	**Change in living conditions**
29	**Revision of personal habits**
30	**Trouble with boss**
31	**Change in work hours or conditions**
32	**Residence move**
33	**Change in school**
34	**Altered recreational activities**
35	**Diminished involvement in church**

(continued)

36	Fewer social engagements
37	Minor financial worries
38	Change in sleeping habits
39	Fewer family get-togethers
40	Change in eating habits
41	Loss of vacation plans
42	Change in holiday traditions
43	Minor violation of the law

*Life events that may be specifically related to chronic pain are in boldface.

stress of chronic illness is particularly debilitating because partners expect to be equal. She writes: "You lose your expected future, first, and then your marital equality."

Often the well spouse must carry an increased workload. In some cases the person in pain simply can't do the tasks that he or she used to do; in others, the pain person needs to spend time and energy seeking medical treatment. The side effects of medications can also mean a reduced energy level for someone in pain, with the result that household chores and errands such as shopping are no longer possible. Although the chores themselves are usually interchangeable (for example, men can fold laundry as well as women, and vice versa), most people enter a relationship with the expectation that their partner is going to carry his or her weight. Well spouses may also have to increase their hours at work, take on additional employment responsibilities, or even obtain a second job if the bills begin to pile up. Invariably, when illness strikes one partner, the dynamics of the spousal relationship change, and the well partner often has to do much more than originally anticipated.

Parenting roles can also change drastically when one parent becomes ill. Raising children is a difficult job even for two committed and healthy parents. For the well spouse of a chronically ill parent, sole responsibility for getting the children dressed and bathed and then attending to homework and chauffeuring duties can be overwhelming. When one parent is not able to participate as actively as in the past, the pain condition not only adds increased burdens to the well spouse, but also takes something important and meaningful away from the person in pain. Both partners suffer as a result. (Chapter 6 discusses childrearing issues in detail.)

In a memoir entitled *Beyond Chaos: One Man's Journey Alongside His Chronically Ill Wife*, Gregg Piburn satirically summarizes his increased workload as a result of his wife's chronic pain.[3] He imagines the following newspaper ad:

> Wanted: Someone to assist chronically ill person with demands of life. Must be dependable, caring and organized. In addition, applicant must be creative, humorous and romantic. Willingness to drop everything to assist in crises is a requirement. Applicant must also be a great conversationalist who knows how to have fun. Counseling skills are a major plus. An emphasis on group and family dynamics is desirable. Prefer Jungian to Freudian school of thought. Advanced first-aid certification is a plus. Must be good with kids, know how to prepare a decent meal, have exceptional housecleaning skills and be great (yet sensitive) in bed. Since this is a part-time job, applicant must also hold down a full-time job. Apply only if willing to make a lifelong commitment.

Piburn effectively uses humor to diffuse what obviously is a difficult and emotionally charged home situation. Humor can be a wonderful tool even in very serious times. Laughter is a powerful antidote to stress and helps us cope in a variety of different circumstances. In all likelihood, there is a physical basis for why laughing is good for us—our bodies release certain chemicals when we are mirthful that may promote healing.

Loss of Intimacy

The loss of a loving and sexually fulfilling relationship is very common in marriages in which one partner suffers from chronic pain. Although this topic is discussed in more detail in the next chapter, it's important to point out here that a loss of physical intimacy can profoundly affect a marriage. In studies and surveys of couples living with chronic pain, as many as 50–75 percent of couples report having little or no sexual contact.

The reasons for the decline in sexual intimacy may be numerous. Obviously, pain itself can be a contributing factor—the person in pain might fear having more pain, and the spouse may worry about inflicting more pain. Men sometimes are unable to sustain an erection because of the pain or medication-related issues. Women might have a decreased sexual interest secondary to the pain, or side effects from medication. A well spouse who is overworked and tired might resent sex as just another chore—one easily avoided. In addition, partners struggling with anger, depression, anxiety, and guilt may have difficulty participating in a loving physical relationship. Even in strong marriages, physical intimacy can be lost when one partner develops chronic pain.

Loss of Financial Status

In *Mainstay*, Maggie Strong has a chapter titled "Downwardly Mobile"—which is exactly what happens to many families when one partner becomes ill. Even if the pain partner is not out of work, the family may experience a loss of wages because of a breadwinner's inability to work overtime, failure to be promoted, or absenteeism owing to doctor's appointments or sick days. Medical bills can also contribute to the financial woes. Even in families that are not experiencing financial challenges, both partners may live in fear that their current situation will worsen if the pain person becomes increasingly disabled. Couples may curtail their usual activities such as dining out or taking vacations in order to pay the mortgage or save for a rainy day. Chronic illness brings uncertainty, and financial uncertainty—or worse yet, the loss of one's usual financial status—can be devastating.

Money is one of the main causes of discord among married couples. Even without the burden of illness, people worry and argue about financial issues. Couples often come to a relationship with individual ideas about earning, spending, and saving money, which can make tackling finances difficult in the best of circumstances. Unexpected financial burdens can strain even the strongest marriages and may destroy marriages that are already unstable. When one spouse becomes chronically ill, both partners can feel angry, resentful, or guilty about the financial problems the family must face. Parents might worry about how money issues will affect their children, and children in turn might blame their parents for not providing them with what they believe they need. As Strong points out, the downwardly mobile spiral in families coping with chronic pain can precipitate a major crisis in a marriage.

Loss of Emotional Balance

The emotional toll that any chronic illness takes on an individual and the family is enormous. In a marriage, the emotional roller coaster can be exhausting. A chronic illness can bring a couple closer together—an illness might unite partners in new ways. For example, couples may work with each other to research treatments or seek out specialists. They may spend more time together at home or going to health appointments. For such couples, the recognition that life is fragile and that they have limited time to be together can spark a more nurturing relationship.

The family brought together by illness is a favorite topic and familiar cliché of movies, television, and popular fiction. This happens in real life, too, but far less often than the opposite—usually families, and in particular couples, face more difficulties in their marriage once someone becomes sick. In some instances, a sick partner changes the focus of the marriage and allows the original conflicts to take a back seat or to resolve. For instance, one of my patients is a middle-aged woman whose husband had been out of work for more than a year. For months, the focus of their marriage had been on helping him deal with unemployment and the associated loss of self-esteem. He was depressed, and they were battling because he wasn't actively seeking a new job. Then, rather suddenly, my patient developed severe low back pain that jeopardized her ability to work. Both partners focused less on his depression and more on her pain, which in turn helped mobilize him to begin actively looking for work. He found a job, and she was able to concentrate on getting medical treatment for her back. The conflicts surrounding his unemployment took a back seat and ultimately resolved when the focus of the marriage shifted from his issues to her medical condition. Of course, the problems in a marriage don't always resolve so neatly. When issues are shelved and partners shift their focus, the relationship may worsen rather than improve. Chronic illness is a delicate balancing act for both partners.

Perhaps the most common emotions that couples must deal with are grief and loss. Elisabeth Kübler-Ross has described the five stages of grief that a dying person experiences. These same emotional stages apply to those persons in chronic pain, though not everyone experiences them all, or in the order that Kübler-Ross lists them. The stages include denial, anger, bargaining, depression, and acceptance. In the first stage (denial), both partners might be thinking that the illness or injury isn't really happening or will be over soon. During the second stage (anger) the couple may be wondering, "Why is this happening to us?" The third stage (bargaining) can involve thoughts such as, "just let me work until I put the kids through college," or "if I go to church regularly, then let this pass." In the fourth stage (depression), the couple must face the fact that the illness is not likely to go away. They must come to terms with that reality before they can move onto the final stage of acceptance. It's only by working through the grief that couples can come out on the other end of the cycle and figure out how to live their lives in a different but meaningful way. Just knowing that the feelings they are experiencing are shared by many people dealing with chronic pain can be a comfort to those in crisis.

The anger stage of the grieving cycle can be particularly destructive to a relationship. Both partners may be angry at the illness itself and wonder why they have been chosen to deal with such a blow. We all question why some people have terrible afflictions while others enjoy good health throughout their lives. There are no obvious answers to this question, and the only thing that we or our loved ones who are struggling with chronic pain can do is rise to meet the challenge.

Partners who are angry at each other often manifest their feelings in a variety of ways (for example, verbal or physical abuse, emotional withdrawal, substance abuse, and so on). Each partner might in some way feel that the other has contributed to the illness or the problems in the marriage. For example, a well spouse may believe that the pain person can participate more fully in sharing the workload. On the other hand, the person in pain may feel that the well spouse is asking too much of him. Both partners often feel angry with themselves, the situation, or each other. Instead of looking to each other for support, they might turn to others. At one extreme, some individuals might turn to extramarital affairs. Others will turn to friends and family members as their primary confidantes. Support groups, whether they meet online or at a local facility, can be invaluable, provided that individuals do not devote all their time and energy to such groups at the expense of leisure, parenting, and other responsibilities.

In relationships where the well spouse has to assume additional responsibilities, he can feel overwhelmed, sad, and even angry. The well spouse may resent the loss of a reliable partner or may just feel sad that the partner can't do the things she used to do. Good times might be in short supply if the pain person doesn't feel well enough to socialize, travel, or even participate in family events. The well spouse might curtail activities such as going out with friends or working out at the gym in order to manage the increased workload. Feelings of isolation may ensue if this results in the loss of friends and people who provide emotional support.

The loss of the original marital equality creates not only a sense of overresponsibility for the well spouse but also enormous emotional challenges for the person in pain. The pain person can also feel frustrated, sad, and angry. Sometimes the emotional imbalance is precipitated by the illness itself, as is the case with women who suffer from conditions that can cause hormonal fluctuations (for example, endometriosis). Illness can easily marginalize someone's role in the family, causing a loss of self-worth and self-esteem. Such a person might become less of an authority figure in the family if many of the decisions about finances, chores, and childrearing are being made by the well spouse. Like the healthy partner, the person in pain might feel increasingly isolated and lonely. It's not surprising, then, that people who have chronic pain and their spouses suffer much higher than normal rates of clinical depression.

It's not uncommon for patients to tell me that they need help from their spouses, but that their partners do too much or too little. This results in anger and resentment, which can cause the patient to retreat emotionally from his or her partner. I am often struck by how much a patient expects from a partner. The person in pain thinks the spouse should know intuitively *exactly* how much help he or she needs. Frequently a visit to my office is the first time a couple discusses what they need from each other.

Chronic pain couples can also experience other emotions such as guilt or fear. Often the diagnosis of chronic pain cannot be medically confirmed the way diabetes or hypertension can. With the latter two diseases, objective tests (blood sugar and blood pressure levels) can be measured and verified. This is generally not the case in chronic pain. Frequently, there is no specific test that can verify the diagnosis, and there probably will never be tests that can accurately measure exactly how much pain someone experiences—regardless of the diagnosis. Given such uncertainty, couples often fear what the future will bring. Well spouses may not believe that their partner has as much pain as she is subscribing to. Pain partners might not feel validated. Both spouses may feel guilty over the situation and their responses to it.

Also complicating this emotional roller coaster is the fact that well spouses are often not so well themselves. They frequently have their own medical problems to deal with. Even if they don't, they are more likely to develop *new* health problems once they have a sick spouse. Indeed, the well spouse might experience enormous stress, helplessness, depression, anxiety, sleep problems, gastrointestinal changes, and even pain as a result of coping with a spouse's chronic illness.

Relationships in Crisis

Studies show that 25–65 percent of individuals in chronic pain relationships note a decrease in marital satisfaction following the onset of pain in one partner. Interestingly, well spouses are more likely than their partners to report that they are unhappy with their spouses and their marriages. When you consider all the different roles a spouse generally assumes, and how those roles may change once someone becomes ill, it's easy to see why couples struggle.

It's difficult to arrive at accurate statistics regarding infidelity in chronic pain marriages, but the number is likely higher than the norm. This is probably true of all marriages in which one person is chronically ill. Chris McGonigle, who "had been raised a 'good Catholic girl,'" writes

*Roles That May Be Altered When One Partner Has
Chronic Pain*

Supportive husband/wife
Mother/father
Breadwinner
Community volunteer
Cook
Gardener
Chauffeur
Errand runner
Homework supervisor
Social director
Disciplinarian
Confidant
Bill payer
Financial planner
Active neighbor/friend
Vacation planner/participant

of her decision to begin an affair in *Surviving Your Spouse's Chronic Illness:* "Of all the things I had imagined myself doing over the course of a lifetime, seeking out another man while I was still married was never one of them."[4] McGonigle writes of her extreme fatigue and desire to resume a semblance of normal life. She calls her husband's chronic illness his "mistress" and writes that it was the first thing he thought about when he woke up and the last thing he thought about when he went to bed.

Indeed, marriage is a difficult bond to keep intact even under the best of circumstances, which explains why approximately half of all marriages in the United States fail. In families in which one person is chronically ill, the divorce rate is significantly higher—perhaps as many as 75 percent of couples end up divorced when one person is sick. Of those couples who stay together, many are unhappy and remain married for reasons such as financial security, religious beliefs, or guilt. One of my patients with chronic back pain who recently went through a divorce confided, "I wasn't the man she married, so she didn't want me anymore."

Healing Relationships

In most cases, chronic pain isn't a life-threatening condition, though often it's a lifelong one. Thus couples are forced to choose whether they will remain together or part ways. Although either path may be fraught with emotional turmoil and great personal sacrifice, there are ways that committed couples can improve their relationship.

If you are the person in pain, it's important to recognize the barriers that are keeping you from having a loving, supportive relationship. Of course, the pain itself may be an issue, but often it's secondary to other things. For example, are you engaging in maladaptive pain behaviors (say, constantly moaning or sighing) that frustrate your spouse? Are you relying too heavily on your spouse to do things for you or to take on responsibilities that were once yours? If so, these are things that you can slowly work to change.

If you're the partner in pain you also need to look inward and assess how you feel about your current situation. Are you depressed, angry, abusive, or reclusive? Do you feel that if you're not healthy, then you're not loveable? Do you feel unattractive? It's important for both partners to understand that people who are chronically ill often perceive themselves differently than their spouses view them. Although you may feel less attractive because of an injury or weight gain, it's unlikely that your spouse sees you that way. Rather, your partner might be feeling a strain in the relationship because of *your* reaction to how unattractive you feel. Examine your relationship and how your own feelings are affecting it. Talk to your spouse about your thoughts and consider professional marriage counseling if the relationship remains troubled.

If you are the well spouse, it's important for you to understand that your loved one is most likely feeling insecure and frustrated. Who wouldn't? Although your feelings may not have changed, the way you express them might have. It's perfectly normal for you to be wary of a spouse who is struggling emotionally—particularly if anger or hostility is present. If your spouse is withdrawn or depressed, it may be hard for you to connect with him or her. You have every right to be exhausted if your spouse is very demanding or you have taken over many new responsibilities. At the same time that you examine the changes in your spouse, look at how you're reacting to them. Are you overly solicitous to demands? If so, remember that spouses who are too helpful may actually encourage more pain and disability in their loved ones. Rather than saying, "Oh, I know you can't do anything, I will do everything for you," encourage your partner to do as much as possible. This leads to increased self-esteem and self-worth. At the other extreme, if you have disengaged from the relationship and are not at all solicitous, your spouse may not feel valued or loved. Reflect on your relationship and how both you and your spouse are handling things. Be open to getting professional counseling if you can't begin healing the relationship on your own. It may take a third party to recognize what you and your loved one could be doing to regain your loving and intimate relationship.

As you examine your relationship and look at all the changes that have taken place, be sure to include both the positive and the negative. It may seem that everything is negative, but with some reflection you will most likely find some potential benefits to your new situation. Perhaps spending more time together will bring you closer; or maybe small things that might once have gone unnoticed now take on new and special meaning. A chronic illness can actually improve your relationship by helping you and your spouse to become more loving and compassionate. You might include the fact that you're no longer able to take things for granted. Perhaps you have acquired new skills such as patience. If you're in a marriage in which both partners are dedicated to each other, chronic pain can provide the opportunity to deepen your commitment and love for each other.

Many of the patients I treat are involved in long-term commitments. I watch them struggle with chronic pain and the challenges it brings to their relationships. It saddens me to see how some marriages and families are torn apart by illness. On the other hand, it is heartening to behold the wonderful ways in which some couples rise to meet the tremendous challenge of living a life that now has fewer options. There is hope for those who are open to reevaluating their marriage and themselves.

There is no doubt that when someone has chronic pain, both partners and the entire family suffer. Many couples are not able to adjust to a new way of life. Help is available. For a list of resources see the Appendix. Chronic pain does not have to rob a couple of everything they hold dear. Instead, it can provide an opportunity for partners to reevaluate their lives and their plans and in many cases make new plans that can be equally fulfilling.

3

Intimacy and Sexual Activity

CHRONIC pain has a marked effect on people's ability to remain intimate and sexually active. This is an issue for both the person in pain and the healthy partner. Although intimacy means different things to everyone, it goes far beyond sexual intercourse. Intimacy is the way that couples relate to each other—both physically and emotionally. Sexuality may involve special looks that couples give each other, verbal communication, caresses, and finally the sex act itself. The respected social worker Mary Romano described female sexuality in the following manner, though her description is equally applicable to men: "Sexuality is more than the act of sexual intercourse. It involves for most [people] the whole business of relating to another person; the tenderness, the desire to give as well as take, the compliments, casual caresses, reciprocal concerns, tolerance, the forms of communication that both include and go beyond words . . . sexuality includes a range of behaviors from smiling through orgasm; it is not just what happens between two people in bed."[1]

A majority of people with chronic pain report reduced sexual interest and satisfaction. In some studies, more than 80 percent of patients and their spouses report significant reduction in or elimination of sexual activity. This is often due to a lack of information about how chronic pain and intimacy are related. For example, many people may not engage in intercourse because they fear it will make their pain worse. Studies show just the opposite; in fact, research shows that very often intercourse is followed by several hours of pain *relief*. Intimacy for most people is a valued and cherished part of a committed relationship with their partner. In order to help regain this special part of a relationship, couples living with chronic pain must explore the reasons behind this loss of intimacy.

Physical Problems

One of the main reasons people give for decreased sexual activity is the fear of increasing the pain or making the underlying condition worse. This can be a legitimate concern. Sexual activity, and in particular intercourse, is physically strenuous and may put pressure on painful joints, muscles, and so on. In most cases, though, couples need only find a comfortable position to experience pain relief rather than an increase in discomfort.

Although it's unusual for chronic pain conditions to lead to *physical* problems with sex, such as achieving and maintaining an erection, this certainly does occur in some instances. As difficult as it may be, patients should discuss problems with erections, ejaculation, vaginal lubrication, and so on with their doctors. Remedies exist for nearly all physical problems causing sexual dysfunction, but the treatment will vary considerably depending on the problem and the underlying condition. One simple way to help determine whether you or your partner is having true physical problems (particularly with respect to erections and ejaculation) is to assess whether the problem occurs all the time or just sometimes. For example, a man who came to see me for his low back pain was very depressed about his inability to perform sexually. He and his wife were having marital problems, and she was angry with him for being out of work because of an injury. He told me that the one place they had always connected in the past was in the bedroom, but now even that was a dismal failure. He did note, however, that whenever they went on vacation and were away from the usual stresses of daily life he had no problems achieving an erection or ejaculating. From his history alone, it was obvi-

Classes of Pain Medications That Can Affect Sexual Function

Antianxiety medications
Antidepressants
Antiseizure medications
Muscle relaxants
Opiates (narcotic medications)

Some Drugs and Medications Associated with Sexual Dysfunction

THERAPEUTIC CATEGORIES	GENERIC NAMES	BRAND NAMES
Antihistamines	Diphenhydramine	Benadryl
Antidepressants	Amitriptyline	Elavil
	Buspirone	Buspar
	Fluoxetine	Prozac
	Citalopram	Celexa
	Doxepin	Sinequan
	Imipramine	Tofranil
	Nefazodone	Serzone
	Nortriptyline	Pamelor
	Paroxetine	Paxil
	Sertraline	Zoloft
	Trazodone	Desyrel
	Venlafaxine	Effexor
Amphetamines	Dextroamphetamine	Dexedrine
Histamine H-2 blockers	Cimetidine	Tagamet
Antihypertensives	Spironolactone	Aldactone
	Clonidine	Catapres
	Guanethidine	Ismelin
	Hydralazine	Apresoline
	Methyldopa	Aldomet
	Phenoxybenzamine	Dibenzyline
	Propanolol	Inderal, Cardinol
	Reserpine	N/A
Anticonvulsants	Gabapentin	Neurontin
	Phenytoin	Dilantin
	Diazepam	Valium
Barbiturates	Pentobarbital sodium	Nembutal
Antipsychotics	Thioridazine	Mellaril
Skeletal muscle relaxants	Baclofen	Lioresal
	Cyclobenzaprine	Flexeril
	Dantrolene sodium	Dantrium
	Diazepam	Valium
Antiparkinsonians	Benztropine	Cogentin
	Trihexyphenidyl	Artane
Anticholinergics	Atropine sulfate	N/A

(continued)

THERAPEUTIC CATEGORIES	GENERIC NAMES	BRAND NAMES
Antianxiety agents	Chlordiazepoxide	Librium
	Diazepam	Valium
	Doxepin	Sinequan
	Hydroxyzine	Atarax
Hipolipidemics	Clofibrate	Atromid-S
Heart failure drugs	Digoxin	Lanoxin
Antivertigo agents	Dimenhydrinate	Dramamine
Obsessive-compulsive	Fluvoxamine	Luvox
disorder drugs	Paroxetine	Paxil
	Sertraline	Zoloft
Antimaniacals	Lithium carbonate	Eskalith, Lithane, Lithobid, Lithonate, Lithotab
Monoamine oxidase	Isocarboxazid	Marplan
inhibitors (MAOIs)	Selegiline	Eldepryl
Narcotics	Morphine	Astramorph, Duramorph, Kadian, Infomorph, etc.
	Oxycodone	Percocet, Oxycontin, Roxicodone
	Codeine	Tylenol #3
	Hydrocodone	Hycodan
Thiazide diuretics	Hydroflumethiazide	Diucardin
	Chlorthiazide	Diuril
Miscellaneous		
Ethyl alcohol		Alcoholic beverages (beer, wine, liquor)
Nicotine		Tobacco products
Psychedelics		LSD
Street drugs		Cocaine, heroin, marijuana

ous that his problems were not physical but rather emotional. Although physical problems with sex can occasionally be intermittent, they don't magically disappear when someone goes on vacation.

Medication side effects are a common reason for decreased sexual drive in both men and women. Medications can also greatly affect the ability of men to have and sustain erections and to ejaculate. For example, many medications that are used to treat chronic pain will result in increased fatigue, which may in turn affect sexual desire. Some medications may also cause or worsen symptoms of depression or anxiety. This, too, can affect one's ability to participate in a physically intimate relationship. Ironically, antidepressant medications, while helping with mood elevation, can interfere with sexual drive or satisfaction. It's also important to note that people who are "self-medicating" with illicit drugs or alcohol can experience significant sexual side effects from these substances.

Deconditioning, or decreased physical fitness, may be another factor in reduced sexual activity. In general, having intercourse with a familiar partner is equivalent to rapidly walking up two flights of stairs (for women the energy expenditure may be a little less, and extramarital, clandestine sex usually requires more energy). But for some people, walking up a flight of stairs or having intercourse may be exhausting or even impossible owing to a lack of exercise and diminished physical stamina. This is usually a reversible problem (unless someone has severe heart or lung disease) and can be addressed with an exercise program that focuses on increasing physical conditioning. Of course, you should consult your doctor before beginning any new exercise regimen.

Finally, if someone is very ill, frequently hospitalized, or recovering from surgery, there may simply be few opportunities for sexual intimacy. Depending on the individual and the medical condition, this situation can improve over time, stay the same, or become even more problematic.

Emotional Problems

Emotional issues have a profound impact on intimacy in all relationships. It's essential to recognize that chronic pain may have nothing to do with marital discord and intimacy. In fact, as with the general population, many couples in which one person suffers from chronic pain have longstanding relationship issues that predate the pain problem. In some instances when the relationship is rocky to begin with, one person may be using pain as a way to ward off intimacy. For example, a wife with an angry and domineering husband might use chronic pain as a reason for not being intimate with her spouse. Or a husband with back pain might cite his condition as a reason not to have sex with his alcoholic wife. When a relationship shows serious problems, it is almost always necessary to have some type of intervention such as professional counseling in order to improve intimacy.

Even in the absence of serious relationship issues, chronic pain couples still can experience reduced intimacy and marital satisfaction for psychological reasons. Someone in pain may be overwhelmed with day-to-day activities and simply too tired to enjoy an intimate relationship. The same might be true of a well partner who is tired from doing additional work to compensate for the ill spouse. This loss of interest may be compounded by medications that exacerbate fatigue. Symptoms of depression and anxiety (common in chronic pain sufferers and their spouses) can also contribute to a lack of interest in sexual activity. Once again, medication side effects may worsen these symptoms. Avoiding sex might also be a way of demonstrating to a well spouse the *authenticity* of the pain in conditions where there is no obvious physical evidence; or one partner may withhold sex or participate grudgingly as a punishment either intentionally or unintentionally. People in pain may not feel attractive or sexy, or they might project their own fears about their diminished appeal onto a partner. All these emotional factors potentially play a role in reduced physical intimacy in couples without serious relationship problems.

Fear of conceiving a child and passing along a chronic disease or having to cope with the responsibility of raising a child while ill can also explain why some couples might not engage in sexual intimacy. In most chronic pain conditions there is no direct hereditary link. Chronic pain does, however, tend to run in families, probably for a variety of reasons, including a predisposition to certain physical characteristics (for example, poor posture, upper body weakness, the early development of osteoarthritis that is associated with aging, and so on) and learned behaviors (for example, a child who watches her mother struggle with back pain may anticipate and then develop the same or similar condition). Never-

theless, the fear of conceiving a child, particularly if that child will be susceptible to a parent's medical condition, may be a factor in abstaining
from intercourse. Couples might also fear the *responsibility* of raising a
child at a time when they are unable to invest the necessary emotional,
physical, and financial resources. A physician who is an expert on a particular condition or syndrome can explain the hereditary risks and how
they may affect unborn children. Couples should also initiate discussions with their physicians about which birth control methods may be
best for them.

We are just beginning to appreciate the prevalence of emotional problems and intimacy issues stemming from childhood sexual abuse in
chronic pain patients. A few preliminary studies suggest a higher-than-
average incidence of self-reported childhood sexual abuse among pain
patients—this is particularly notable in women who suffer certain types
of chronic pain, especially chronic pelvic pain that occurs without an obvious underlying physical problem. The relationship between a history of
sexual abuse in someone with chronic pain and subsequent sexual dysfunction as an adult is not well understood. What we do know is that in
the general population, people who have been sexually abused as children have a higher incidence of psychological and social dysfunction in
adulthood.

Sometimes the emotional reasons for reducing or avoiding sexual intimacy are not entirely obvious to the partners involved. For example, anger can play a role in fostering poor relationships. One partner might be
angry with the other for a variety of reasons—and neither one of them
may realize it. Feelings of frustration, anger, and disappointment often
contribute to emotional barriers that inhibit intimacy. The pain partner
may feel as though the well spouse is too demanding or not sympathetic
enough. The well partner might feel cheated out of having a healthy
spouse. In addition, either partner may fear rejection when initiating or
engaging in sexual activity. Intimacy, by its very nature, places people in a
vulnerable position. Individuals in pain are frequently worried that they
have gained weight or that they are not as physically attractive as they
were prior to the onset of their pain condition. They may feel less con-
fident than they did as a "healthy person." Moreover, concerns over the
inability to perform physically in order to satisfy a spouse can lead someone to disengage and not even make the effort.

Fostering Intimacy

For most couples, improving intimacy and sexual relations is an achievable goal. As noted, professional counseling is essential in relationships where there is spousal abuse, alcoholism, or other serious problems. Even in less dire circumstances counseling can provide a valuable tool for addressing emotionally charged intimacy issues. For more information on how you can find a trained healthcare professional who can provide appropriate counseling, ask your doctor for a referral or check the resources in the Appendix. It's important to seek counseling only from professionals who are experienced and qualified in the area of sexuality. There are many "sex therapists" who aren't legitimate. Your doctor and the organizations listed in the Appendix can help you find a qualified expert.

Intimacy can also be improved when both partners understand the pain person's medical condition and specific restrictions. Coexisting medical conditions can cause sexual dysfunction, and it's important for both you and your partner to understand how these conditions might be affecting your ability to be physically intimate. If you're not sure about a specific medical condition, ask your doctor for advice. If positioning is an issue (as it often is for people who are in chronic pain), consult guides that address the problem (see the Appendix). Intercourse in a comfortable position has enormous psychological rewards and can provide pain relief as well.

Intimate relationships can also improve with such basics as regular exercise, proper nutrition, restful sleep, and taking pride in your appearance. It's important to use alcohol sparingly and to avoid illicit or "recreational" drug use. A bigger bed, strategically placed pillows, and a firm mattress can also promote comfortable intimacy. Furthermore, recognizing that intercourse need not be spontaneous and unpredictable to be enjoyable can be helpful. In fact, planning a romantic interlude early in the day when both partners feel less fatigued can rekindle intimacy. The timing of medications can often be worked around this planned encounter. Also, understanding that intimacy involves much more than sexual intercourse can go a long way toward healing a relationship. A gentle massage, soft caress, or loving kiss can be extraordinarily meaningful.

Common Physical Conditions That May Interfere with
Sexual Function

MEN

Arteriosclerosis
Low testosterone levels
Parkinson's disease
Prostate problems
Spinal cord injuries

WOMEN

Decreased estrogen level
Prolapsed uterus

BOTH MEN AND WOMEN

Alcoholism
Arthritis
Bowel or urinary incontinence
Cardiovascular disease
Chronic pain
Dementia
Depression
Diabetes
Hypertension
Infections of the genitalia
Multiple sclerosis
Respiratory disease
Stroke
Thyroid problems

Proper medical treatment directed at easing the pain will make intimacy and life in general more bearable. Physical therapy to improve mobility, increase endurance, and reduce pain can also be useful. It's wise to do a medication review with your doctor to optimize pain relief without causing undue fatigue or symptoms of anxiety and depression. Some people find that hot packs or cold packs used at home both before and after intimate encounters help relieve any discomfort. Finally, there are medications and other treatments for physically based sexual problems (Viagra being just one of them). Your doctor should be able to discuss the various options with you or refer you to someone who has expertise in this area. Despite the high incidence of intimacy problems in chronic pain couples, committed partners have a variety of options to significantly improve their sexual relationship.

4

Work Issues

THE U.S. economy loses billions of dollars each year to employment issues stemming from chronic pain. But these financial statistics, though impressive, mask the real suffering that occurs when someone who provides financial support to the family is affected by chronic pain. Medical studies have mainly focused on chronic low back pain, which is the most common injury-related reason that people lose time from work or become totally disabled. Yet despite the sparseness of literature in other areas of pain, a great deal can be extrapolated from what we have learned about workers with chronic low back pain. For example, we know that direct medical costs (for physician visits, surgery, medications, and so on), while expensive, grossly underestimate the social and societal costs from decreased work productivity and the retraining of injured workers. We also know that there are significant indirect costs to the family when the primary provider has been injured and is out of work. These costs may include an increase in emergency room visits for children who are no longer receiving routine preventive medical care because the family has lost its healthcare benefits. Or they may include additional services from the public school system in the form of psychological counseling or tutoring for children who are doing poorly in school because of stress at home.

Unemployment also brings with it the loss of a social life with coworkers and diminished prestige for the worker and the family. Coworkers who are unaware that a colleague is struggling to remain employed despite constant pain may suspect malingering, resulting in a loss of respect or career momentum. Thus chronic pain affects more than the wallets of working people and their families.

Compensable versus Noncompensable Injuries

The idea of receiving compensation for an injury dates back to ancient times. The Tablet Nippur No. 3191 (2050 B.C.) and the code of Hittites (1300 B.C.) both provided for monetary recompense for various injuries. In India during the first millennium, extensive laws were written regarding compensation for bodily harm, which generally meant punishment of the perpetrator. For example, kicking someone could be punishable by amputation of the foot and punching by amputation of the hand. These early traditions paved the way for more sophisticated compensation laws that have become commonplace in many countries.

Today's compensation laws were primarily shaped in response to how we now work. The development of automated machinery in the 1700s and 1800s dramatically changed the way people did their jobs. Instead of laboring in a small shop or out in the fields at their own pace, many people began working in large factories and had to keep up with the machines. The hours were long and the work was often dangerous and hard. By 1900, it was not uncommon for someone to work in a factory for ten to twelve hours a day, six days a week, for meager wages. The unionization of labor, which really began in the second half of the nineteenth century, came about as a way to ensure adequate compensation and safe working conditions.

Workers' compensation laws are now fairly standard in most industrialized nations. But with compensation has come a dramatic increase in the number of injured-worker claims. Moreover, studies have consistently revealed that in situations in which people are compensated, they tend to report more injuries, have worse pain and disability, and remain out of work longer (or not return at all). Thus, the system is far from perfect. The fact that people who are injured can get compensated for their injuries means that they might be influenced in a negative way—healing may be delayed or not occur at all because of factors that have more to do with money than with medicine.

The two most common situations in which an individual may be compensated for an injury are in the workplace or in a motor vehicle accident. When young doctors rotate through my practice, I instruct them to pay close attention to the course of someone's injury and observe whether it is a compensable injury. For example, in any given week it's not uncommon for me to see three men (or women) with similar low back sprain or strain-type injuries. Typically, the man who injured himself in his own yard shoveling snow will return to work very quickly (this is a noncompensable injury), whereas the man who was injured at work and the man who was hurt in a car accident will take much longer. Even if they all receive the same treatment and their injuries are nearly identical, very often there will be a significant difference in their return-to-work dates.

In my practice, nearly every person injured in a motor vehicle accident walks in the door having already seen a lawyer—even if the injury only happened the day before. Time and time again, patients have told me that they don't want to return to work because their lawyer has told them they'll get more money in the settlement if they remain out of work. So despite my telling them that they are physically able to go back to work, they remain disabled. The same is often true for people I see with work-related injuries—particularly those who are involved in litigation. It's important to note, though, that this delay in returning to work does *not* mean that someone is faking an injury. What it means is that someone who has suffered a noncompensable injury has a lot of incentive to go back to work in order to continue supporting the family *despite* having pain. By contrast, someone who has suffered a compensable injury has another option (that is, to stay at home and still receive a paycheck or some other compensation at a later date from a settlement) that is often more appealing than returning to work. Compensation adds another level of complexity to healing an injury for both the physician and the patient.

Work Injuries

More than 80 percent of us will suffer from low back pain at some point in our lives. In fact, low back pain is second only to upper respiratory infections (colds) as a reason people give for taking sick time from work. Each year millions of workers sustain low back injuries on the job and billions of dollars are spent in both direct medical costs and indirect costs such as lost time from work, administrative expenses, and employee retraining.

Not surprisingly, the people most likely to suffer work-related injuries are those who do the most physical labor—especially heavy lifting. The three occupations with the highest injury rates are materials handlers, truck drivers, and nursing aides. Other occupations with high injury rates are maids and heavy laborers, including construction workers and carpenters. Sedentary workers are also at risk for low back injuries and overuse injuries from repetitive activities such as using a computer keyboard. These overuse injuries have various names including cumulative trauma disorders or repetitive strain injuries.

Perhaps surprisingly, the level of pain an individual experiences is usually *not* a good predictor of whether he or she will report a work injury or go out on disability as a result of an injury. Although it's often hard to predict what will happen in individual cases of work-related injury, there are some interesting patterns. For example, in 1986 the journal *Spine* published a series of reports from a large work-injury study done at the Boeing Company.[1] According to the results, workers who stated that they "hardly ever" enjoyed their jobs were 2.5 times more likely to report acute back injuries than workers who stated that they "almost always" enjoyed their jobs. Other studies have confirmed that unhappy workers are both more likely to report an injury and less likely to return to work following an injury. The level of autonomy that a worker has also appears to make a difference in whether she returns to work. Employees who enjoy a lot of autonomy (for example, they can set their own pace and avoid activities that make their pain worse) are more likely to return to work than those with little autonomy. Workers with low levels of education are also more likely to stay out of work after an injury. This may be due in part to the fact that such workers often have more physically demanding jobs and fewer options for switching to another type of work.

A number of other factors can affect someone's return to work after an injury. These include whether the person's job is physically demanding and whether he has the option of modified duty or "light duty." Studies have shown that the longer someone is out, the less likely that employee is to return to work. For example, the vast majority of people who suffer back injuries return to work within a month. But of people who are out of work for six months, only 50 percent will return to work; after twelve months only 25 percent will return; and after two years, the rate drops to just about zero. Research has also shown that psychosocial factors can play a role in the likelihood of someone's returning to work. Least likely to return are people who have poor English proficiency, people who are angry at their employer, and people who are involved in litigation. A history of previous injuries, illicit drug use or prescription medication abuse, and poor cardiovascular fitness are also risk factors for a delayed return to work.

Compensable Injuries and Litigation

Compensable injuries often go hand in hand with litigation. Compensation laws vary from state to state, and individual companies often have complicated compensation policies of their own. To the uninitiated the bureaucracies may be overwhelming, and so they may seek legal counsel just to help explain the nuances of the system. This is particularly true for people with limited education and few work alternatives. The difficulties associated with trying to figure out how to get compensated might add to the injured person's feelings of powerlessness. Some people become frustrated with what they perceive to be a system that cares more about the paperwork than about helping people who are legitimately hurt. They may hire a lawyer in part to "make the system pay" for their suffering. For a small percentage of people who are injured, the condition may be so physically devastating and the compensation needs so great that litigation is the only way to resolve the claim.

Nick, a patient of mine, experienced what in all likelihood was an unavoidable nasty legal battle following a work-related injury. Nick was a custodian at a mall who was asked to come in on his day off when the shopping center flooded after torrential rains. Nick used the proper equipment, a "wet vac," to get rid of the water; however, the machine malfunctioned and Nick was severely electrocuted. His injuries were truly catastrophic—he was paralyzed and suffered a traumatic brain injury that left him with permanent cognitive deficits. He lived with tremendous post-electrocution pain, which is common in these types of injuries. In this case, Nick sued the manufacturer of the machine that malfunctioned for several million dollars in order to cover his medical bills and living expenses for the rest of his life. After several years of litigation, the case was settled out of court for significantly less than he was suing for but well over a million dollars. These types of catastrophic injuries almost always require litigation in order to reach what both parties view as fair compensation.

Regardless of why someone chooses to litigate a claim, the process is sure to be stressful for the individual and the entire family. Many people don't realize before beginning litigation how it will actually work. In truth, there are many different scenarios that can take place, and most of them entail serious hardships for the family. For example, an injured employee who receives money every month from workers' compensation benefits may find that the checks stop once litigation starts; indeed, it's not unusual for an employer to halt all benefits until the litigation is resolved. The legal process can take several years, during which time the family has to make do without this income. There may be significant costs associated with the litigation as well—especially if the attorney is not hired on a contingency basis, whereby he or she gets paid a certain percentage at the conclusion of the case. The injured party must be aware that some attorneys who are supposed to have their clients' best interests at heart may be biased when it comes to litigating injury-related claims. Since attorneys usually make more money the bigger the settlement, and settlements are typically larger the longer someone has been out of work, then it makes sense from their perspective to counsel their clients to remain out of work—especially when their clients are suffering from chronic pain. But this is very often not sound advice from either a medical or a financial perspective.

Another one of my patients, Bob, spent nearly three years unemployed after a work-related back injury. He was clearly unable to return to his job as a truck driver since it entailed a lot of heavy lifting; however, he could have gone back to work almost immediately after his injury in a more sedentary position. Bob was fired from his company, and throughout the time I treated him, he was in litigation with his former employer. He came to see me every one to two months for more than two years and every single time he would come in, I would recommend that he look for a job that was part-time and sedentary. Bob would leave my office and discuss this with his lawyer, who would tell him that if he returned to any type of work, he would get less money from his lawsuit. So for nearly three years Bob remained out of work and became increasingly depressed. Finally, I sat down with Bob and did the math. His lawyer was hoping for a settlement of $100,000. If Bob was lucky enough to get this much money, he knew that one-third would go to his lawyer right off the bat. That would leave him with around $67,000. He had approximately $30,000 in unpaid medical bills, so after those debts were paid, Bob would be left with $37,000. By that time, Bob had been out of work for three years, so I told him that if he had worked part-time for the past three years he would have had to make just a little over $12,000 each year to equal what he might get from his settlement. After I reviewed the actual numbers with Bob, he went right out and found a job as a bus driver for the elderly. Bob made nearly $25,000 per year working part-time, and his job did not worsen his chronic back pain. Moreover, his spirits immediately lifted once he found himself in a job where he was appreciated and needed. His lawyer settled the case for significantly less than he had hoped, and Bob realized that he had wasted three years of his life listening to a lawyer who not only did not care about his psychological well being but also cost him tens of thousands of dollars in income that he could have earned if he had returned to work shortly after his injury.

Often in injury-related litigation the family as well as the injured person is under surveillance. It's not unusual for companies to hire a private detective to help determine whether the claimant is truly injured and to what degree. Nor is it unusual for family members to be subpoenaed and forced to testify about a loved one. I was recently involved in a case in which the defendant's insurance company subpoenaed and deposed the injured man's girlfriend, with whom he had lived for several years. The line of questioning focused almost exclusively on their sex life, since part of his claim was that the chronic pain he was suffering impacted every aspect of his life, including his physical relationship with his girlfriend. The transcript from this deposition was startling in its invasiveness into their personal life. The girlfriend was asked questions about how often they had sex, what positions they used, where they had intercourse, whether her partner achieved orgasm, and so on. This particular deposition was humiliating for her as well as for the injured man, and it's now a matter of public record.

The legal arena can play havoc with what is already a difficult time by making the person in pain and the family feel hopeless. The situation can be particularly demoralizing when employers imply that the injured party is somehow at fault or, worse yet, "faking it." But of course there's another side to the litigation problem. As noted, evidence supports the fact that the more injured people are paid for being out of work, the greater the number of claims and the longer the duration of the claims. When an attorney is involved litigation may take even longer. In the medical literature, mitigating factors in injury compensation claims that go beyond the physical injury are often referred to as "secondary-gain" issues, which in this context basically means that someone who is injured may not return to work as soon as possible if there is the chance that compensation will be forthcoming.

Occasionally, of course, someone really will exaggerate his or her symptoms in order to remain out of work while at the same time receiving compensation. I remember one case of a police officer who was shot in the leg. The officer's leg was healed and all the physicians who treated him were convinced that he had no significant residual effects. Yet he refused to return to work. We concluded (in part on the basis of surveillance tapes to which we had access)—and I believe to this day that we were correct—that he was simply scared rather than suffering from any significant pain. This officer had good reason to be scared—he worked in a particularly dangerous neighborhood, and there was a decent chance that he would be shot again, perhaps fatally. Nonetheless, from a medical perspective, there was no reason he could not go back to his job. I'm not certain of the end result of this litigation, but I seriously doubt that the officer was successful in his lawsuit.

Disability and Unemployment

Despite the prevalence of worker-compensation claims, the vast majority of people with chronic pain remain gainfully employed in their usual occupations without specific job accommodations. Yet some people, in order to remain employed, require a certain amount of flexibility at work. In 1990 the Americans with Disabilities Act (ADA) made it illegal for employers to discriminate against individuals with disabilities, including chronic pain, as long as they could perform the *essential functions of their jobs with or without reasonable accommodations*. The heart of the ADA is that employers must provide "reasonable accommodations" for employees who have a disability and require some type of assistance or special equipment in order to continue working. The law was designed to level the playing field, and in fact the ADA defines reasonable accommodations as "changes to the work environment or the way in which tasks are customarily performed to enable an individual with a disability to enjoy equal employment opportunities." Reasonable accommodations can vary greatly, but they might include a reduced workload, or a piece of equipment such as a telephone headset for someone with a neck injury. One of my patients who has a congenital amputation of one arm and who recently had shoulder surgery on her intact arm requested voice-activated software as a reasonable accommodation in order to be able to use her computer without using her injured arm. Another one of my patients took her company to court (and won) because the employer refused to provide a handicapped parking space as a reasonable accommodation. I always advise my patients to use the term "reasonable accommodation" in any written communications with their employers, and I always use that language when I write letters on behalf of my patients.

In some instances, there are no reasonable accommodations that will allow someone to continue working. For example, one of my patients, a college professor, sustained a shoulder and knee injury in a car accident. Unfortunately, she also suffered a brain injury that left her with symptoms of short-term memory loss and an inability to concentrate. In this case, there were no reasonable accommodations that would allow her to function as a college professor owing to her cognitive problems. Another patient who worked in construction fell off a roof and injured his back. After undergoing a series of operations, he was unable to return to a job that involved a lot of heavy lifting, bending, and climbing. In both of these scenarios the patients have two choices. The first is to undergo vocational retraining. The second is to apply for total disability (meaning they are completely disabled—usually for life) through work (if the injury is work-related), through a private disability insurance policy (if they have one), or through the government (Social Security Disability Insurance or Social Security Income).

I always try to encourage people to seek vocational retraining rather than total disability, whenever possible. For most of us, work is an important part of who we are and how we view ourselves. People who become totally disabled and don't return to work often lose their self-esteem and social support system; they also face serious financial hardship. Whereas financial difficulties will affect the entire family in obvious ways, loss of self-esteem and sense of purpose in a partner or parent can be equally devastating for the whole family. Vocational retraining is frequently an option if someone is willing to invest the time. The cost of meeting with a vocational counselor and undergoing retraining will usually be paid by either the employer or a private company (if the injury was work-related) or by a government agency that is dedicated to providing vocational guidance and counseling. Most vocational services are funded by the federal government (the United States Department of Health and Human Services) and channeled to state vocational agencies. For more information, contact the Council of State Administrators of Vocational Rehabilitation (see Appendix). The agency names vary from state to state, but they are similar in their mission, which is to restore disabled individuals to the highest level of employment of which they are capable.

Psychological Effects

The poet Ralph Waldo Emerson once said, "As soon as a stranger is introduced into any company, one of the first questions which all wish to have answered is, 'How does that man get his living.' He is no whole man until he knows how to earn a blameless livelihood." My husband and I learned the value of a man's work when we decided that he would stay home to raise our children. At first we were astonished at how differently newly introduced acquaintances responded to him now that he was a stay-at-home dad and no longer an Assistant United States Attorney. As a man without a job, he was easy to dismiss—and people did so regularly. The truth is that, for better or worse, we are judged by who we are and what we do. Thus people who are unemployed, for whatever reason, are at a distinct disadvantage in social environments.

Being both disabled *and* unemployed is a kind of "double jeopardy." To suffer not only from physical pain but also from the effects of society's disregard and in some instances disdain is an incredible burden for anyone to bear. It's no wonder that both men and women who have chronic pain and are unable to work have high rates of depression. Chronic pain sufferers who are unemployed also appear to be at a higher risk of contemplating suicide than those who continue working. This is not surprising when we consider that the highest rate of male suicide in the twentieth century was during the Great Depression, when people couldn't find work. Although both chronic pain and unemployment are risk factors for suicide, other factors that may contribute to a higher rate include a history of past suicide attempts, known history of depression and/or substance abuse, single status without strong family support, and lower socioeconomic status.

Stress on the Family

When a breadwinner in the family has chronic pain and is unable to work in his usual capacity or at all, the entire family is radically affected. Family members may experience great stress at no longer being able to count on a once-dependable adult to function as he traditionally has. They may be uncertain about whether the family will be able to afford the lifestyle to which they are accustomed. For example, the children may wonder, "Will we have to give up our home?" or "Will my parents be able to afford to send me to college?" The well spouse may have to consider returning to the workforce, working overtime, taking on a second job, or looking for a higher-paying job.

As noted, litigation is an extremely difficult and stressful process. Many people are not prepared for the fact that they may be under surveillance and that the entire family may be surreptitiously videotaped. One of my patients was filmed on a cruise ship after his children pitched in to send him and his wife on a vacation. His lawyer argued that sitting on a cruise ship where people waited on him was no indication that he was able to return to work. But judges and juries tend to have little sympathy for people whom they view as "living the good life" while at the same time seeking compensation because they claim they are unable to work. This is why many lawyers counsel their clients to avoid doing anything that will raise red flags in a lawsuit—with the result that some people with chronic pain do even less than they are able to do. Thus when a young child asks Daddy or Mommy to play outside, she may get consistently turned down because of ongoing litigation.

Bob became increasingly depressed over the three years that he was out of work. His wife complained that he was unresponsive to her needs and only thought of himself. His children didn't understand why their dad didn't laugh or play with them anymore. One time Bob told me money was so tight that on a trip to the grocery store he had to tell his children that he couldn't afford to buy them the candy bars they begged him for. He had cried on the way home. Bob asked me, "What kind of man can't buy a candy bar for his kid?" Although it might seem like a trivial thing to deny a candy bar to a child, the constant deprivation and change from the former standard of living take their toll on the family. The attitude of the person in pain also dramatically affects how the rest of the family is able to cope.

If you or your partner are out of work because of chronic pain, familiarize yourself with various employment-related issues. Know that pain does not necessarily preclude someone from working. It's important to seek legitimate medical counsel about when it's appropriate to return to work and under what circumstances (for example, with vocational retraining or modified duties). You should also understand the pitfalls associated with compensation-related injuries—especially when they are litigated. Families need to consider what's best for everyone involved and how they can all function optimally given the current situation.

5

Childbearing and Inheritance

Maria was a young woman in her early thirties with a history of chronic low back pain and migraine headaches whom I had been treating for a number of years. Maria had deferred getting pregnant until her pain was managed enough to be tolerable. The only way it was bearable, however, was with the regular use of medications that could potentially harm an unborn baby. When Maria decided she was ready to have children, we had several frank discussions about childbearing and inheritance issues. These included the following points: (1) Would her child be susceptible to migraine headaches (possibly) and chronic low back pain? (not necessarily); (2) Could she take her current medications (no) or alternative medications? (yes, but in very limited amounts); (3) Would her pain worsen while she was pregnant? (the migraines would likely improve and the back pain would likely be more problematic as the pregnancy progressed); and finally, (4) Could she go back on her current medication regimen when she was nursing? (no, but she would have more choices of medications than when she was pregnant).

I hadn't seen Maria for several months when she came in with a beautiful new baby boy. She reported that her migraines had in fact disappeared while she was pregnant and that her back pain had stayed about the same until the last couple of weeks, when it had worsened. At that point, like most women in the final stages of pregnancy, she was generally uncomfortable and had a variety of aches and pains. Maria never felt discouraged because she was too excited about the arrival of her baby. She was caught up in decorating his room, going to baby showers, and making plans with her husband. Labor went smoothly as well. Maria had discussed various pain control options with her obstetrician prior to going into labor and together they had agreed that an epidural would be appropriate midway through labor. Maria came back to see me after the baby was born for advice about how to get back in shape and how to manage her pain while she was nursing. She was the happiest I had ever seen her.

Although Maria's story is a successful one, similar experiences are not unusual among people with chronic pain. Of course, things could have turned out much differently, which is why it's so critical for anyone with a medical condition to discuss with their doctor issues surrounding inheritance and childbearing. There are many factors to consider, and the more informed you are, the better equipped you will be to make the right decisions for you and your family. In this chapter I provide an overview of some of the issues you might want to discuss with your spouse. I'll also suggest some topics you should discuss with an obstetrician or other physician who is involved in your or your spouse's care.

Heredity

The question in almost every scientist's mind is not *whether* genetics plays a role in illness but *to what extent*. As we come to understand diseases and their genetic influences, we search for knowledge about how to modify these factors in order to ameliorate or even cure some medical conditions. Science has made enormous strides in the past decade in understanding the relationship between disease and heredity, so much so that the future never looked brighter when it comes to changing how we perceive, treat, and prevent many illnesses.

Chronic pain is certainly influenced by genetic factors, but we're still exploring the extent to which genes (nature) play a role versus the environment (nurture). There's no space here to discuss the many different underlying diagnoses associated with chronic pain, but some examples of diagnostic conditions that cause chronic pain and clearly have a genetic component are familial hemiplegic migraines, which are five times more common in family members than in the general population, and endometriosis, which is more frequently diagnosed in women who have family members with this condition. Other chronic pain conditions may have significant genetic factors, but the relationship is not as evident. For example, there are many environmental reasons someone might have chronic low back pain, including working as a heavy laborer, sustaining an injury in a car accident, having poor overall fitness owing to a lack of regular exercise, or being significantly overweight. Any one of these environmental factors can be a plausible explanation for someone's chronic low back pain. Yet we can't rule out genetic reasons for chronic low back pain either. For instance, is someone who is overweight genetically susceptible to this condition? Is a driver who sustains a back injury in a car accident more physically vulnerable than the passenger who wasn't injured? Are some people more genetically sensitive to pain than others? When it comes to chronic pain, we are only beginning to understand how nature and nurture work together. Most likely both contribute to chronic pain, but probably to different degrees depending on the underlying medical condition, the individual's genetic makeup, and the environmental influences.

Reproduction

Chronic pain conditions can affect conception in a variety of ways. For example, *fertility* refers to the ability to conceive a child, whereas *fecundity* is the likelihood (or probability) of conception. Women with rheumatoid arthritis are usually able to conceive (they have normal fertility) but it takes longer (fecundity is affected) than average. Hormonal fluctuations in some medical conditions can potentially affect fertility. Intimacy itself may be a factor in conception as the rates of couples engaging in sexual intercourse decrease dramatically when someone has chronic pain. Medication use can also influence reproduction—either because medications can interfere with the biologic process of conceiving a child or because women (in particular) defer getting pregnant while on medications out of fear that they might harm an unborn baby. If you have concerns about having a baby, talk to your doctor. He or she should be able to provide you with information and even a referral to a fertility expert if appropriate. With all the new treatments available for infertility, couples who are experiencing problems have numerous options. In many cases, however, treatment for infertility is not covered by medical insurance, and it can be quite costly.

Chronic pain can also affect the *desire* to have a child. Both women and men who suffer from chronic pain might consciously decide *not* to have children because of their medical status. For example, studies of women suffering from severe forms of juvenile rheumatoid arthritis (JRA) note a reduced wish to have children. Some people may decide to defer the decision while they are actively seeking medical care. Other couples may idealistically think that a child will improve their lives and make up for other losses. Deciding whether to have children is an important decision under the best of circumstances; when one partner suffers from chronic pain, the decision can be especially difficult. If you or your spouse has a chronic pain condition, sit down together and carefully consider your specific situation and how the illness might impact the child and the entire family. I always encourage patients to talk candidly with their doctors in order to be as well informed as possible. You'll certainly want to know if the condition has a heritable component; if it will worsen during pregnancy or afterward; what the long-term prognosis is; if medications will affect the unborn baby; and so on. The more information you have, the better able you are to make these life-altering decisions.

Planning whether or not to have children is a very important decision. But sometimes people with chronic pain might unexpectedly find themselves pregnant for the usual reason—unprotected sex. Some women in chronic pain might forgo contraception altogether because they don't want to take yet another pill or because their doctors advised them against taking oral contraceptives (although there are many alternatives to "the pill," some women might not use anything if they decide this popular option isn't right for them). Both men and women suffering from chronic pain may not engage in sexual activity on a regular basis, and so they may not plan for contraception as they would if they had sex more frequently. It's important for everyone to use contraception or some alternative type of pregnancy prevention method unless they are *planning to conceive*. Otherwise they might well have to deal with an unexpected (and often unwanted) pregnancy.

Planning for conception means not only deciding you want to conceive a child, but also becoming informed about the effects of the medications you or your partner (particularly the mother) are taking on the unborn baby. Any medications that might be harmful should be discontinued prior to conception. Many people are not aware that even simple anti-inflammatory medications can affect an unborn child. For example, some anti-inflammatory medications (when taken by the mother) have been shown to interfere with kidney function in the fetus and potentially decrease the amount of amniotic fluid (the fluid in which the baby is suspended). "Natural" remedies such as herbal preparations can also have serious effects on the fetus. Moreover, women should begin taking prenatal vitamins containing folate *before* becoming pregnant.

If you or your loved one is suffering from chronic pain and you have questions about conceiving a child or about how *not* to conceive a child, then you should have a discussion with your doctor as soon as possible. These are very important issues, and your doctor should be able to answer all your questions or at least refer you to someone who can. It's especially critical that you talk to your doctor right away if you find yourself with an unexpected pregnancy.

Pregnancy and Labor

Pregnancy causes profound physical changes in *all* women, so it's no surprise that it especially affects women with chronic pain. What might be surprising is that some women actually experience a marked *reduction* in their pain and other symptoms while they are pregnant. For example, with both multiple sclerosis and rheumatoid arthritis, symptoms generally improve during pregnancy. Once the pregnancy is over, though, the usual symptoms typically return. In these two conditions pregnancy generally makes things better for a while, and, even though the diseases become more active postpartum, there doesn't appear to be any worsening of the symptoms overall compared with prepregnancy. Migraine headaches are another example of a chronic pain condition that usually improves during pregnancy.

Unfortunately, improvement during pregnancy is not typical of most chronic pain conditions. Although there aren't a lot of studies on chronic pain and pregnancy, we do know that more than one-third of *healthy* women experience back pain during pregnancy. Women with pre-existing back pain are more likely to experience the same or worsening pain because being pregnant puts enormous stress on the spine and soft tissues surrounding the spine. On the other hand, a number of my patients with low back pain happily went through pregnancy despite having their usual or even worse pain. For some women, physical pain is tolerable during pregnancy because the end result—a much-wanted child—is so satisfying.

Special considerations during pregnancy and labor will depend on the underlying medical condition. For example, women with low back pain may feel better with a corset as the pregnancy advances. In women with scoliosis, special delivery procedures such as a cesarean section or vacuum extraction might be necessary. If you are pregnant or considering becoming pregnant, discuss these issue with your obstetrician as they pertain specifically to you and your medical needs.

In general, labor can be improved with good coaching and emotional support, massage, the presence of a supportive partner, and upright positions and hydrotherapy (bathing) during the early stages. Conventional anesthesia can also help with labor pain and contractions. If you have chronic pain, discuss pain control options with your obstetrician before you go into labor. Your doctor should be able to give you specific advice on the use of medications to control labor pain as well as such things as when bathing is helpful, for how long, and at what temperature.

Breastfeeding can be problematic for some chronic pain conditions for a number of reasons. First, women who nurse their babies have restrictions on the medications they can take because drugs are secreted into breast milk. Second, some women, such as those with neck or arm pain, might have difficulty holding their babies while nursing. Third, elevated hormonal levels that occur in breastfeeding in some instances might have an effect on disease activity (for example, prolactin may be associated with increased arthritic activity in rheumatoid arthritis). You may elect to breastfeed for a time and switch to formula, supplement breast milk with formula from the outset, or breastfeed exclusively. Debates about breastfeeding can be politically charged, and there certainly are proven benefits to nursing (the primary one being that antibodies from the mother are transferred to the child, providing initial protection from various infectious diseases), even if for a short period of time. But remember that this is a *personal* decision. If you have questions about what to do, discuss them with both your child's pediatrician and your treating physician.

Although we don't fully understand the exact role of genetics versus the environment in most chronic pain conditions, there's a lot of good information available to help you consider childbearing and inheritance issues. Your pain doctor, family practitioner, obstetrician, and child's pediatrician are all good resources. In some instances, you might be referred to someone who specializes in genetics if there are serious concerns about inheritance issues for a particular medical condition. Keep in mind that though you might feel a little awkward initially, it's never too early to begin discussing these important subjects with your doctor or doctors.

6

Growing Up with a Parent in Pain

A FEW years ago a woman came to see me after being injured in a car accident. For several months she had been experiencing severe neck pain and headaches. During her evaluation and subsequent follow-up appointments it became clear that her family was suffering at least as much as she was. My patient was almost exclusively in charge of raising her two young children as well as taking care of things on the home front. Her husband, who had been raised in a traditional home, resented that his wife was not able to do all the household tasks as she had before the accident, and he refused to pitch in to alleviate her burden. Several times she came to my office in tears, often towing her five-year-old son along. As her physical symptoms gradually improved, her psychological state deteriorated. Despite having less pain, she became increasingly depressed and overwhelmed. Unfortunately, she rebuffed my suggestion that she see a mental health professional because she thought psychotherapy would bring shame to herself and her family. During one January visit, her son was chatting amiably with me and I asked him what Santa had brought him for Christmas (I knew the family celebrated Christmas from previous conversations we had). The little boy's face crumpled and he began to cry. I looked to his mother for an explanation and she said, "Santa didn't bring him anything this year because he was bad."

I was stunned. I couldn't believe that any mother, even a mother in chronic pain suffering from depression, would deliberately inflict such trauma on her child. For years I was angry with this patient of mine—my heart ached so much for the child that I had a difficult time giving her the compassionate care that I pride myself on delivering. She eventually left my practice, and it wasn't until I sat down to write this book that I thought about what happened in that family. Clearly there were some serious problems, and probably not all of them stemmed from the mother's car accident. But I believe that the chronic pain this mother suffered tipped the scales and led this family into a downward spiral.

My patient was probably like a lot of mothers—struggling to do the right thing by her children and making minor mistakes as she went along. Then one day a car slammed into her car and her life changed instantaneously. Coping with debilitating pain, she went from doctor to doctor seeking relief. When she wasn't making doctors' appointments, she was pursuing accident-related issues with her lawyer. Between her pain and her medical and legal issues, she became increasingly overwhelmed. Her uncooperative husband wasn't much help, and she felt unable to ask for support elsewhere. Her young son saw all of this and knew something really bad had happened. But no one attempted to explain it to him; what they did tell him left him confused and bewildered. Think what it must have been like for him to have a mom who was always angry and sad and a dad who was withdrawn and resentful. Of course he began to act out—he didn't have the information or the tools to deal with the situation. Whereas before he had been a nice, well-mannered child, he now became filled with rage. He withdrew from his mother and consistently pulled "stunts" to attract the attention he craved (and draw the focus away from his mother). My patient, already overwhelmed, did the only thing she knew how—she disciplined him unmercifully.

As I write this, the little boy is in his teens and on the verge of adulthood. I am sure that the legacy of his mother's chronic pain has affected him profoundly. I can only hope that at some point the family got the professional counseling they needed. But I suspect they struggled on on their own, and instead of making the usual childrearing mistakes that every parent does, they fell into the category of deeper dysfunction. But it needn't be that way. A parent's illness can bring hardship and crisis to the family, but there are ways to help children cope with this situation. Most parents probably understand that they ought to be open and honest with their children, but they might be unsure what to say or how much to tell them, how to explain confusing medical terms and, in the case of young children, the abstract concept of chronic pain.

Parents who want to protect their children may inadvertently fall into a pattern of dishonesty. But the truth is, whether you're honest with your children or not, they'll most likely figure out what's going on. The problem with leaving them to their own devices is that their understanding of the situation is often inaccurate. All of us at times let our imaginations run away with us, but children, with their limited understanding of the world, can't put things in the proper perspective without parental guidance. If you have chronic pain and have not talked to your children, they may be imagining that you're dying. If they carry that thought a little further, your children may be wondering if they'll be given up for adoption. They may think that your pain is their fault and that it might happen to them, too. Your children may sense tension between you and your spouse and assume that you're planning to get a divorce. Or they may just feel a sense of dread and not really be able to come up with any firm answers. Whatever the case, having a truthful discussion with them is certainly better than letting them jump to their own conclusions.

At a minimum, parents should share the following information with their children:

1. *Tell them the name of your condition.* All children should be told the name of the condition you have as best you can describe it. Sometimes the condition can only be described as chronic pain syndrome rather than a specific diagnosis such as migraine headaches. But it's important to put a name to the problem.

2. *Tell them why you have the problem.* Explain to your children why you have pain. If it occurred because of a car accident or some other trauma, then tell them so. If there are things that you don't understand or for which there are no clear answers, then tell them this, too.

3. *Give details about what you expect to happen now and in the future.* Explain that you're getting help from your doctor and that although you may have to live with pain for a long time, or even forever, you are trying new treatments that you hope will help. If there are noticeable side effects, explain them.

4. *Explain how your condition affects your moods and ability to participate in activities.* Children need to know what to expect from their parents. So tell them what you can and can't do—especially as it pertains to family routines and special occasions. Let your children know that your love and devotion to them are unchanged despite all the time you now spend go-

ing to the doctor or otherwise dealing with the pain. Explain that your moods are not their fault and that you're working to become emotionally stable. Stress that you're still their parent, despite your condition.

The amount of detail children need to know varies depending on their age, maturity, and ability to understand the explanation. In order to give a general approach, I have categorized children into three basic stages: the Very Young Child, the Older Child, and the Adolescent Child. These are arbitrary categories that are meant to give readers a general idea of how to approach their children at different ages. So though you should always be honest and open with them, the specific details you give them will depend on what you think your children are ready to hear.

At the onset of your condition, use your best judgment and tell them what you think they can grasp. Then bring the subject up again every few weeks or when something significant changes about your condition (for example, you have surgery or some other procedure). This approach keeps the lines of communication open and gives your children the opportunity to ask you additional questions.

The Very Young Child

Children in this category include toddlers and preschool-age children. When dealing with this age group, begin with just the essential details. You can use dolls or stuffed animals to help the child understand where you have pain. This "play technique" is very effective in young children. You may also use words they understand such as "boo boo" rather than more technical terms.

Because children this age are involved in "magical thinking," that is, they often believe that just by thinking something they can make it happen, it's important to tell them that they didn't do anything to cause Mommy or Daddy to be sick. Stress that even if they get mad at you or they don't do what they're asked to do, they are not responsible in any way for your pain. Also, explain that they are not in danger and that they will not "catch" your condition (this is usually the case with chronic pain conditions, but if your situation is different, it's important to be honest). Last, explain that you're not going to die, give them up for adoption, or otherwise abandon them. If your child has not voiced concerns about these issues and you don't want to scare him, you can reassure him in a loving way by saying something like, "I will live a long life and be here to take care of you just like I always have."

Choose a calm time when your child isn't tired or hungry and pick a setting without too many distractions. You may not be able to do this all in one sitting. That's fine—it's important to consider your child's attention span. If you need to stop because your toddler's attention has wandered or your preschooler is squirming, then bring up the subject at another time when you think your child is ready to hear more. Keep in mind that children in this age group often can't fully comprehend or remember even the simplest details, so you may have to repeat yourself several times.

Additionally, you can anticipate that whatever you tell your child will likely be repeated—possibly inaccurately. One of my good friends is a pediatrician who contracted strep throat three times one winter. Her two-year-old daughter repeatedly told people that both she and Mommy had a sore throat. Several neighbors didn't want their children to play with her daughter (although the little girl never had strep throat herself) because they erroneously believed that she was infected and contagious.

The Older Child

School-age children will be able to understand more about what's happening in your family. Once again, start with basic information such as the name of your condition, why you have it, and what you expect to happen now and in the future. Simple diagrams and explanations from books and websites can help. Also, stress that your pain is not their fault and that they can't catch it from you. Once you've provided this information, give more specific details about what's happening in your family. Who's going to take care of this child's needs? Who will drive him or her to school, help with homework, make the meals, and so on? Ideally, you want to change family routines as little as possible, but often change is unavoidable. *The important thing is to let your school-age children know how things are going to change and how they will be affected.*

If you require ongoing medical treatment, you might consider bringing your child along to a doctor or therapy appointment. This would give her the opportunity to ask questions and to learn more about what's going on. School-age children should be told something about your prognosis. It's important to explain that your illness is a chronic condition that you will not die from (unless, of course, you have terminal cancer or another condition where you do have a shortened life expectancy—in this instance, you should work with a professional counselor to decide the best way to impart the news of a poor prognosis). If you and your doctor believe that your symptoms will improve with treatment, then share that news with your child, but once again, be honest. It's always better to say that you're not sure than to tell a child something definitely will happen when it may very well not.

Carrie is a ten-year-old girl whose mother has multiple sclerosis. Although her mother has chronic pain, her main symptom is vertigo. The family rarely discusses the mother's illness, and Carrie has learned to equate dizziness with such feelings as anger and frustration. Carrie would thus complain of dizziness whenever she became upset or worried. Once the family's pediatrician pointed this out to her parents, they were able to talk to Carrie more openly about her mother's condition and about her feelings. Consequently, she no longer complains of vertigo.

The Adolescent Child

Adolescents have a much greater understanding of medical problems than younger children, but the information they have may not be very accurate—especially if it's gleaned from the media. Parents who are confused about their own health conditions can sometimes pass along inaccurate information to a child. Samantha is a fifteen-year-old girl who has never had any significant health problems. One morning after staying up late studying for an examination she awoke with a stiff neck. Her mother, who suffers from chronic neck pain, immediately assumed that her daughter had suddenly developed the same neck condition that she has. After rushing to the pediatrician's office, both Samantha and her mother were immediately reassured that this was not the case. Samantha had simply strained her neck by bending over her desk for hours the previous night, and her symptoms resolved in a few days. It was good that Samantha's mother sought professional help right away, rather than unnecessarily worrying herself and her daughter.

Because adolescence is a time when young people begin to form their own identity and establish independence, chronic pain in the family can be especially confusing. An adolescent may feel torn between newfound autonomy and the need to stay close to home during a crisis. Adolescent children are ready for very detailed explanations. All their questions should be answered as honestly and completely as possible. If the illness is causing tension in the family, bring this up. It's important to give adolescent children the most realistic explanation possible and to tell them what is expected of them.

Ideally, adolescents should have someone outside the immediate family circle in whom they can confide without feeling selfish or disloyal. Moreover, because adolescence is usually a time of great emotional turmoil even for young people with healthy parents, children in this age group should be carefully watched to see whether they might need additional help from a professional counselor.

How to Tell if Your Child Needs Help

A number of warning signs may indicate that your child needs professional help in dealing with his or her emotions and current situation. It's crucial that children of a chronically ill parent receive adequate professional help as they struggle with the day-to-day issues within the family. Successful treatment almost always focuses on the whole family. Parents who see their children become casualties of their illness feel guilty and depressed, and consequently experience more pain than parents who take an active role in promoting good mental health and coping skills for their children.

Mood Changes

As your family struggles with issues surrounding chronic pain, there will of course be times when family members feel glum or worried. In children, the time to worry is when these moods become *persistent or are present more than they were in the past*. We all have a baseline mood level that fluctuates as events happen in our lives. When good things happen, we feel happy and when bad things happen we experience sadness. Children, too, have a baseline mood level that depends on their individual personalities. The warning sign to look for is a persistent *change* in your child's mood. If you notice such a change, seek professional help for your child.

New or Exaggerated Behaviors

It's important not only to assess your child's mood but also to look for new or exaggerated behaviors. For example, you should be concerned if your usually outgoing child suddenly becomes withdrawn, or if your child begins to act out at home or at school. If your daughter is usually neat but begins to obsess about keeping her room clean, then this could be a warning sign. The opposite is true as well. If your child usually needs prompting to bathe but now completely disregards personal hygiene even with your reminders, then you should consider whether this child may need some counseling. You know your children better than anyone else, so you are the best judge of whether they have troubling new behaviors or exaggerated pre-existing habits that should be addressed by a professional.

Sleep Problems

In my home state of Massachusetts, all children must pass a statewide examination in order to graduate from high school. When children from a school that has consistently ranked among the highest on the exam were interviewed, I was struck by what they reported. I had expected the children to say that they studied hard, but I was wrong. Instead, they said that they were given little homework, and that their teachers encouraged them to sleep ten to twelve hours each night. The moral of this story is that the importance of sleep should never be underestimated.

Sleep problems take various forms depending on the age of the child. Most parents know when their children are having sleep problems—particularly when the children are getting up at night. Another sign of sleep disturbance is sleeping too much. If your child usually sleeps ten hours at night but suddenly can't get out of bed in the morning and wants to nap right after school, he may be clinically depressed. You should seek professional help if you're unable to address the sleep issues successfully.

Increased or Decreased Appetite

An increase or decrease in appetite may signal problems for a child. At the same time, though, change in appetite may also be part of a normal growth stage. This can be confusing for parents. If you're worried, watch your child's mood for signals—be watchful not for a skipped meal here, or the dinner of pizza and ice cream there, but for bigger patterns over weeks and months. Is your child gaining more weight than would be expected at this stage in development, and given his activity level? A sudden increase in frequency and intensity of exercise, fascination with the bathroom scale, and sudden penchant for looser clothing should all be watched and set in a wider context of behavior and mood. Almost all kids (and adults for that matter) exhibit food quirks, but *new* quirks or an obsession with the calories as opposed to the nutrients in food (for instance, counting the calories in breath mints; eating artificial sweetener from the packet as a snack) are highly suggestive and probably cause for concern. In the absence of other worrying behaviors, a child is the best regulator of what he or she eats, and parents are wise to carefully pick their battles when food is the issue. If your child is overeating, then encourage him to exercise. This has powerful benefits in promoting good health as well as improving mood. But if your child is developing significant eating problems, get help sooner rather than later—particularly for teenagers, who are prone to serious eating disorders such as anorexia and bulimia, though these diseases can occur in preteen children as well.

Poor School Performance

My brother is a high school counselor who makes it his personal mission to confront kids who are performing poorly in school. He makes a list of students who need intervention. Most of these students wouldn't be motivated to seek him out, so he goes after them. One by one he calls them into his office and gives them a stern but compassionate lecture filled with the hard facts about the future that awaits them if they don't finish high school. The statistics are alarming—the majority of people who don't graduate from high school live at the poverty level.

One of the most important things to convey to your children, regardless of their age, is the importance of doing well in school. Despite whatever is happening at home, they need to know that you expect them to continue to work hard at school. They need to know that you want them to focus on school and not on you. *They need your permission to keep academic work a priority above and beyond the family's needs.* You need to relieve them of any guilt they may have about spending time on their studies rather than on you or the family. Similarly, school must also be a priority for the parents; you or your spouse need to monitor homework assignments and academic performance and also attend parent-teacher conferences just as you always have. Talk to your spouse and figure out a plan for how to stay involved in your child's school life despite living with chronic pain. Guiding your children in the right direction is one of the best things you can do for your health, because it alleviates stress and gives you something positive on which to focus.

How well your children are performing at school is usually a good indicator of how they're doing in general. Even children who act out at home will likely weather adolescence unscathed if they continue to display resilience and do acceptable work in school. On the other hand, children who begin to perform poorly in school are at risk for significant problems in the future. As a parent you should take this behavior very seriously.

Suicide

It's impossible to describe the devastation families undergo when one of their members, especially a child, commits suicide. The grief and guilt are a burden few parents can bear. In retrospect, there are usually clues that a child was at risk. Experts agree on four signs that should be reason for concern: (1) when a child tells you that life is no longer fun or worth living; (2) when a child talks about dying or killing himself; (3) when a child begins to take risks (for example, getting speeding tickets or being involved in multiple car accidents, behaving in a sexually promiscuous manner, or experimenting with drugs); and (4) when a child attempts suicide, even if the attempt seems overly dramatic and a manipulative bid for attention.

Parents must keep the lines of communication open with all their children—regardless of age. Furthermore, children need to have their feelings validated. They need to be *listened to*. It's imperative that parents not ignore early warning signs in children by dismissing their concerns with responses like, "Oh, your life is just fine. You shouldn't feel that way." Or "Things will get better, just don't worry about it." In particular, parents must take seriously any suicidal behaviors in their children and seek counseling from a professional.

It's hard to help your children when you're experiencing physical and psychological pain yourself. As a parent, you must be honest with your children and tell them what's happening. Give them a realistic idea of the future and what they can expect. Allow them to explain and voice their feelings by asking them questions. Stay in tune with what's happening to them at home and at school. And finally, seek professional help when you feel that your children are falling into a pattern of high-risk behavior that persists despite your best efforts.

7

Chronic Pain in Children

W HEN I was a doctor in training, I spent a lot of time in the neonatal intensive care unit tending to sick and often premature babies. I was told, and I believed then, that these babies did not feel much pain since the nerve pathways that carry pain signals to their brains were not fully developed. This is probably not true—at least there's no convincing evidence that it's true. In fact, recent studies that involve monitoring facial expressions, movement, crying, and other responses to pain in babies and young children have revealed that they may actually experience more pain than adults do under similar circumstances. Such studies have prompted the medical community to rethink the experience of early childhood pain, but we still have a long way to go before we fully understand the effect of pain on children.

Although the literature on childhood pain is sparse, research studies have shown some important results. For example, the vast majority of children who suffer from chronic pain have close family members (often a mother or a father) who also live with chronically painful conditions. This may be true for a number of reasons. We know that some diseases have a hereditary component. In addition, parents who are invested in the medical system themselves might be more likely to take their children to doctors. And finally, it's a well-known fact that children mimic adult behaviors; thus children who see their parents in pain may develop painful conditions and associated pain behaviors (for example, grimacing, moaning, or walking with a limp) simply because they learned this behavior from their parents.

Without realizing it, parents can actually encourage their children to develop chronic pain problems or can exacerbate an already existing chronic pain problem. They can do this in two ways. The first is by being overly sensitive. This behavior usually begins early in childhood with a parent who is exceedingly concerned about the child's physical comfort—always checking to see whether he's covered by a blanket or is wearing enough layers of clothing. The overly concerned parent rushes to the child's side every time he trips instead of reassuring him that a minor bump or scrape is not a big deal. This over-sensitivity to the child's physical comfort can encourage him to become exquisitely aware of even the slightest physical discomfort. It also teaches the child that for any minor physical problem he will receive a lot of attention, and so the way to get attention is to complain of physical pain—whether or not it exists.

The second pitfall is the other extreme—the parent who does not validate and take seriously a child's pain complaints. The parent who does not appropriately comfort a child when she has an injury sends the message to the child that she's not important. This lack of validation of a child's very real experience has detrimental effects. It confuses and angers children. They know they're hurt, so why doesn't Mom or Dad pay attention? Why don't they care? To avoid encouraging pain behaviors in their children, parents should strive for an appropriate level of intervention and responsiveness.

Research has also revealed that children and adolescents who have chronic pain experience more emotional distress than their peers, including anxiety and depression. Similarly, young people with chronic pain have been shown to have lower self-esteem and more behavior problems than other children. Interestingly, the severity of pain is not necessarily predictive of whether children will experience these other problems. *In fact, what seems to influence children more than any other factor is how their parents cope and teach them to cope with chronic pain.*

Why Children Are in Pain

All children are familiar with the acute pain associated with shots at the doctor's office, skinned knees, sore throats, and bug bites. Others will have more serious injuries such as broken bones or lacerations that require stitches.

Many children are also acquainted with chronic pain, which in childhood can take many forms. It can be due to an ongoing serious illness or condition such as sickle cell anemia, juvenile rheumatoid arthritis (JRA), or cancer. In these conditions, the pain may be constant but wax and wane in intensity, as is the case with more severe forms of JRA. Or it may be intermittent, as when a child with sickle cell anemia experiences a sickle cell crisis. Chronic pain can also result from repeated treatment-related procedures in serious medical conditions (for example, leukemia) such as obtaining blood samples (venipuncture), spinal taps (lumbar puncture), or bone marrow aspirations.

Even children who are not seriously ill might experience chronic pain from headaches, stomachaches, earaches, or various musculoskeletal injuries. In these cases, the pain usually occurs intermittently, as with migraine sufferers, who usually have long headache-free periods and then intense episodes of pain when a headache occurs. Dental work and orthodontia can also cause chronic pain for a period of time. In children who are competitive athletes, chronic pain may result from a single ongoing musculoskeletal condition (say, back pain) or from a series of injuries (for example, sprained ankles, knees, or wrists).

A thirteen-year-old girl who is a very high-level competitive ice skater came to my office with her mother. Mom did most of the talking. She explained that her daughter was in chronic pain from a series of ankle sprains. The girl practiced skating for four hours every day after school. She also played soccer, and in fact that's how she got most of her ankle sprains. It was clear to me after examining the skater that she had too much flexibility in her feet and ankles in certain directions and not enough flexibility in other places—this was causing her to roll over on her ankles and repeatedly sprain the ligaments. Appropriate treatment for repeat ankle sprains such as hers includes anti-inflammatory medications, icing the injured ankle, wearing an ankle support, obtaining shoe orthoses (which can be placed in skates and soccer cleats) to better position the feet, and attending physical therapy to improve flexibility and strength. It also involves avoiding activities that aggravate the injury while the healing and rehabilitative process is under way. But because this girl was an elite skater, described by her mother as someone who "someday may go to the Olympics," her mother refused to follow my advice and allow her daughter to take a short break from training. Two weeks after ignoring my advice, the girl once again rolled over on her ankle and this time fractured the bones in the lower part of her leg. This injury sidelined her for much longer than she would have been out if her mother had agreed to follow my original recommendations. Interestingly, when I asked the girl (out of earshot of her mother) whether she was disappointed at not being able to train, she replied that she was delighted to have a rest.

Not all children have parents who push them as hard as this mother, but many child athletes are nonetheless prone to chronic injuries and therefore chronic pain. They may sustain an acute injury (such as an ankle sprain) and either not allow it to heal fully before returning to play or not undergo any rehabilitative measures to keep the injury from recurring. Other children are at risk for the same types of overuse injuries that are common in adults. These injuries may be due not only to overuse of a particular part of the body but also to poor training techniques. For example, although cross-training (as when swimmers run to increase their endurance and give their arms a rest, or runners cycle to build up their lower extremity muscles and take a break from the pounding that goes along with running) has been shown to increase fitness and strength and help avoid injuries, coaches often do not employ this excellent training technique with children.

How Children Understand Pain

The Very Young Child

This age group includes children from birth to preschool age. Because the pre-verbal child is unable to vocalize where it hurts, parents must look for clues of discomfort. As children begin to talk, they can better communicate their pain or at least the fact that they have pain. Even so, it's impossible for children in this age group to be logical about their experiences. They understand things very concretely, and they believe that whatever they experience is obvious to others. For example, a three-year-old who falls down without any obvious injury may exclaim, "Put the Band-Aid right there where it hurts! Can't you see it?" Children in this age group typically have fantasies and believe in "magical thinking." They may view pain as a punishment for an action or even a thought they had. Very young children also believe that their parents have total control (that is, the ability instantaneously to make everything better). If they develop chronic pain, they may assume that their parents are angry with them and that they are being punished. They may think that their parents could instantly take their pain away but choose not to.

Parents may not recognize pain in a child this young. This was the case with two-year-old Joey, who pulled his mother's coffee pot down and sustained second- and third-degree burns over 25 percent of his body. He spent several days in the intensive care unit on morphine and then was discharged to home with Tylenol with codeine. One week after his burn, his mother took him to the pediatrician and reported that he was "clingy." She didn't know what was wrong. She thought that perhaps he had an ear infection. The pediatrician watched Joey during the visit and noticed that he hadn't moved at all—very unusual for a child of this age. She immediately recognized that he was in severe pain, and she admitted him to the hospital for pain control. As soon as he was properly medicated, he began to move and was no longer seeking constant physical comfort from his mother. In the preschool-age child, changes in behavior are often more important than what the child is able to communicate about his pain.

The Older Child

As children reach school age, they become less egocentric and more logical. They begin to understand and describe their pain. By the time they enter school, most children have a limited understanding of the word *pain* and what it entails. Their reasoning is generally based on direct observation, and they tend to be very concrete rather than abstract. Children in this age group typically describe pain as "a sore thing" or "a thing that hurts." They believe that a person who is ill goes to the doctor and gets well quickly. Chronic illness or pain is confusing to them.

In addition to being more logical, school-age children are also increasingly aware of how their bodies function. They are curious and interested in understanding what's happening to them. They also begin to be aware of peer pressure and the fact that people may tease them for being "different." They want to fit in with their peers, and most children this age with chronic pain will recognize that they have a unique problem to deal with. This may cause them some distress and anxiety.

But school-age children do have significant gaps in their knowledge and may have problems coping when they're in pain. Gretchen is a seven-year-old girl who suffers from growing pains—a fairly common problem in children ages six to ten, accounting for between 8 and 11 percent of musculoskeletal pain in this age group. Gretchen has the classic history of pain in both legs that awakens her at night and improves with reassurance, massage, and ibuprofen or acetaminophen. These episodes happen periodically and may be absent for weeks or months at a time. One night after a long pain-free period Gretchen woke up crying hysterically. Her mother reacted as she normally did, by giving her a massage and reassuring her that this episode of growing pains would be over soon. When she tried to offer Gretchen her usual medication, however, the girl became even more agitated and insisted that she didn't like the medication and that it didn't work. Her mother immediately realized that her daughter didn't remember taking the medication for this problem. Once Gretchen calmed down, her mother reminded her that she did in fact like this medication and that it had helped her in the past. Children in the throes of a painful episode may not be amenable to treatment that will likely help them; for this reason I recommend that parents talk to children about their condition during pain-free periods when they are better able to focus.

The Adolescent Child

Adolescents are able to generalize, reason deductively, and comprehend abstract ideas. Their definition of pain is generally more refined than younger children's, and when asked to describe what pain is they will typically respond with something like, "a physical sensation that occurs when the nerves are injured" or "something physical or psychological that hurts a person." Adolescence is a time when teens are excessively focused on their bodies and how they look and perform. It's a time when the "herd mentality" is at its height and children want to be like their peers. For better or worse, adolescents are harshly judged by their peers, and the need to fit in becomes a primary consideration. The teenager who has chronic pain, particularly if he or she has a condition that is physically obvious to others, may suffer dramatically during adolescence. Even if the condition is not apparent, there may be a stigma associated with reporting to the nurse for medications.

Despite their intelligence and increased maturity, adolescents who live with chronic pain often lack the perspective that comes with experience. Parents of adolescents who have chronic pain conditions may also lack perspective, because they are not experiencing the pain themselves or because they may not fully understand the illness and the treatment possibilities. Rosa is a fourteen-year-old girl who was born in Brazil and was diagnosed with juvenile rheumatoid arthritis at an early age. According to the American pediatrician who began treating her when she was twelve years old, neither the patient nor the family ever reported this diagnosis, and in fact, on the initial intake form they had checked off that she did not have any history of arthritis. Yet Rosa lived in chronic pain, and her knees became such a problem that she slept most nights on the couch because she couldn't climb the stairs to her room. When her pediatrician noticed her limping during a routine office visit, Rosa and her mother admitted that she had JRA. Apparently in Brazil Rosa's father had had to give her a series of penicillin injections that left both father and daughter traumatized. The family had implicitly agreed not to mention the JRA for fear that she would again be subjected to a harsh (and ineffective) treatment regimen. Unfortunately, because Rosa and her parents did not explore other treatment options, she suffered far more than she needed to.

Depression is not uncommon in this age group in general, but the risk is heightened for adolescents who live with a chronically painful condition that may be disfiguring. Adolescents with chronic pain often have difficulty keeping up with their peers physically or academically, depending on what condition they have and how it affects their energy level and strength. Poor grades are closely linked with low self-esteem. Teenagers who are not doing well in school or who simply can't keep up physically with their peers will often feel rejected by their classmates, leading to social isolation. They might opt out of situations that are difficult for them (for example, they might cut class or avoid participating in extracurricular activities).

Peer pressure can drive many teens to try alcohol or drugs, and adolescents who are dealing with chronic pain can be particularly susceptible to substance abuse. They may participate in drinking or illicit drug use as a way to fit in with a certain group of people. Depressed teens might see drugs or alcohol as a way to alter their mood and to feel better about their situation. Teens, like adults, might also use these substances to "treat" their pain. All parents of adolescents should be concerned about the possibility of their children using drugs and alcohol, but parents of children with chronic pain should be particularly vigilant.

How Parents Cope with Children in Pain

As parents, we go to extraordinary lengths to protect our children from harm. Parents whose children suffer from chronic pain might feel extremely guilty about their inability to keep their children "safe." They may wonder, "Is there something I could have done to help my child avoid this?" or "Did I wait too long to take him to the doctor?" Guilt-ridden parents often assume that they're responsible for their child's ill health. They may ask themselves, "Is this my fault? Did I make my child genetically vulnerable, or did the way I cared for my child cause this to happen?"

Some parents are disappointed in their sick child—either because she is not "perfect" or because they believe she can and should behave better *despite* the condition. Having a child with chronic pain may bring behavioral challenges parents don't have to face with their other children. The child in chronic pain might be impulsive or angry. He may not accept the medical treatment offered and may display disruptive, aggressive, or defiant behavior. A child in chronic pain is frequently demanding and often tries to dominate the parents' attention, leaving other family members, especially siblings, without the attention they need. All these factors can put enormous stress on the individual family members and their relationships with one another.

Helping Children in Pain

Helping children cope with chronic pain requires parents to be sensitive, compassionate, and at times unyielding. As discussed earlier in this chapter, overly solicitous parents can promote poor coping mechanisms in their children. These young people are at risk for developing maladaptive pain behaviors such as groaning, grimacing, wincing, limping, and so on. On the other hand, parents must be careful not to underestimate a child's pain. Acting as if the pain is no big deal and as if the child should just "deal with it" is not helpful. This approach simply encourages a child to be frustrated and angry. It can result in poor coping behaviors such as acting out in school or lashing out at siblings. Reaching the perfect balance of concern is often an unachievable goal, but being aware of the pitfalls of either extreme can help parents help their children cope with chronic pain.

When dealing with a child who has chronic pain, parents and healthcare providers must recognize the relationship between pain and behavior issues. Pain can be a way for children to gain attention or to avoid unpleasant situations. Parents might be frustrated with how a child is behaving or performing in school. They may recognize that the child is using his pain to seek attention. Some parents make the situation far worse with their own behavior; the mother or father who cringes, gasps, or cries out when the child has a procedure only increases that child's anxiety and pain. A parent who dreamed of an outgoing, accomplished child may subconsciously or consciously have trouble embracing a child who is introverted, hypersensitive, and avoids activities that bring on pain. The child's pain may bring out feelings of exasperation or impatience if the parent believes the pain is used to avoid work, school, or family activities.

An overweight teenage girl recently came to me with low back and leg pain. Her physical examination and x-rays were normal. The pain was worse when she was under stress, particularly when she had to go to gym class, which she despised. During one visit she asked her father to leave the room so she could talk to me alone. He grumbled and made a sarcastic remark but then left. The girl immediately began to cry. She told me that her father constantly made fun of her weight and criticized her for being clumsy. She told me that one time while walking in a parking lot she was nearly run over by a car. Her father had yelled to the driver, "Make way for the elephant; she'll hurt your car more than you'll hurt her!"

Obviously, in this case much more than just the girl's physical pain needs to be addressed. The fact that she feels ungainly, unattractive, and unwanted is in large part due to her father's abusive behavior. She most likely has real physical pain, too. But if her situation at home were different, she probably would not be so *disabled* by her pain. Before she was even old enough to drive, she had begun what will likely amount to a lifetime of seeking out compassionate doctors to reassure her that she's a worthwhile person who deserves to have someone listen to her. Moreover, she had given up on participating in any athletic activities, her grades were poor, and she was battling depression. This is an obvious case of emotional abuse, but even subtle messages that parents may un- wittingly give their children can significantly impact their ability to cope.

Perhaps one of the most important things parents can do to help their children deal with chronic pain (aside from avoiding abusive or even subtly negative behavior) is to be honest with them. Secrecy makes chil- dren feel worried and ashamed. Honesty allows them to accept what's happening to them and allows parents to keep the lines of communi- cation open. Parents need to know what's bothering their children and children need to be reassured with the facts. Of course, honest commu- nication should be age-appropriate. A three-year-old with a life-threaten- ing painful condition such as cancer doesn't need to hear everything about the illness and prognosis, but nothing that is said should be un- true. As children get older, they'll need more information and should be given increasing responsibility for their condition (for example, they should learn to follow whatever treatment plan their doctors have recom- mended). Children also deserve to know what's going to happen to them. If a child is going to get a shot, don't say that it won't hurt. It will hurt—at least for a moment. Similarly, avoid inaccurate euphemisms. For in- stance, the shot will not feel like a "pinch"; more likely it will feel like a "sharp prick." The words you use should of course depend on the age of the child, but the bottom line is that honest, open communication is im- portant at all ages.

All children, regardless of age, want to be in control of their bodies and their environment. Giving children who have chronic pain some control over their situation can provide much-needed reassurance. For example, allowing a child who is going to have a procedure to choose the site for the procedure (for example, asking, "Where would you prefer to have the shot, in your right or left arm?") will provide a distraction, since the child has to concentrate on making a decision, and will also make the child feel more in control of the situation. Another example would be to allow a child to decide when she wants to take her medication (for example, "Would you like to take it now or after lunch?"). Parents can also help their children gain some control by asking them what will help in a given situation. A question such as, "When you're having a headache, what seems to help the most to make you feel better?" will usually encourage the child to behave in a positive manner.

On the other hand, too much control at too young an age can have a negative effect. For example, telling a teenager to go to the doctor alone and figure out what to do to treat his pain without parental guidance and supervision is not appropriate. Moreover, while it's a good idea to give a child some control, it's *not* a good idea for that child to become *controlling*. For example, you should not allow a child to use her pain as a way to avoid unpleasant situations. As a parent, you'll need to set some limits while at the same time exhibiting concern for what might help the child. For example, you might say, "I know you're hurting today, but you still need to go to school. What do you think would help you to feel better while you're at school?"

There is no perfect way for a parent to deal with a child who suffers from chronic pain, just as there are no perfect parents. But we do know that children with chronic pain are best helped by parents who acknowledge their pain and limitations but at the same time firmly encourage them to continue to participate in school and other activities. As children grow they become more independent, but at all ages parents have enormous influence on how their children learn to cope.

8

The Extended Family

I was sitting in a meeting at work one day when there was an abrupt knock on the door. One of my staff members rushed in and hurriedly whispered in a colleague's ear. We all knew it was bad news; this colleague's young husband had just had a kidney transplant, and this was her first week back to work after caring for him following his surgery. Her face turned pale and she left immediately. Before she made it home, her husband was taken by ambulance to the nearest hospital with severe abdominal pain. He had a bowel obstruction that required emergency surgery. We all rallied, sending them meals and covering her patients so she could be with him.

My colleague's husband recovered and is now doing well. But his story is a classic example of an emergency that can't be anticipated. We have all experienced times like these—someone we love gets sick and friends and family become immediately available to help in any way they can. We channel our anxiety and worry into working together—rearranging our lives to assist the person who is ill. This is particularly true when a loved one has a sudden and serious, possibly even life-threatening, medical condition.

But what happens when someone has chronic pain? What happens when there is no emergency situation (or it is long over) and instead there is just a loved one suffering from an illness that is ongoing, hard to define, impossible to see, and without a known cure? Of course most of us have experience with diseases that are hard to see—we know people who are battling cancer or fighting infections, and we believe without question that they are suffering. But let's face it, chronic pain is different—it moves in like an unwelcome guest and refuses to leave. Pain is a subjective experience whereas cancer and infections are much more objective. There are tests that can clearly measure the presence and spread of cancer and the type and extent of an infection. Pain, per se, is not measurable in an objective way. We can measure strength and range of motion of the joints and perform imaging studies (x-rays and MRIs) to determine how much cartilage is left in a joint or how much a herniated disk in the back is pressing on a nerve, but none of these objective tests accurately quantifies pain. When loved ones have chronic pain, it's often not obvious that they're ill. We must take their word for it. And we must believe in this thing that we can't see and don't understand.

Moreover, since chronic pain, unlike many other conditions such as cancer, doesn't have a beginning, middle, and end (usually there's either a cure or the cancer progresses until death), it's hard for friends and family to respond as they ordinarily would in a crisis. People want to see their loved one cured from an illness or recovered from an injury. When that doesn't happen, the usual rules don't apply, and very often they have to charter new and unfamiliar territory. This can be particularly difficult when extended family members and friends are not privy to all the details surrounding the illness. They may find it hard to respond in an appropriate and helpful manner when they don't understand why the person they love is in pain and why the pain is persisting. Misunderstandings can develop and bad feelings can fester when extended family members do not fully comprehend the situation. At the same time, this need to know must be balanced with the sick person's right to privacy.

How the Family Can Make Things Worse

Extended family members might be afraid of appearing callous, inconsiderate, or uncaring if they don't offer to help, but often they don't know what to do. They may worry that they won't know what to say or that what they say will be misconstrued. Their offers to help may be rebuffed if the person in pain doesn't want to let them into her "inner circle." A vicious cycle of wanting to help and not being able to can reinforce negative behaviors in extended family members. At one extreme, a family member might be overly solicitous and smother the person in pain. For example, a mother may give up all her outside activities in order to care for her grown son who has a family of his own. This can create enormous resentment among the immediate family members who want Dad/Husband to resume his role as caregiver. The man's siblings may feel that they or their children are being ignored by their mother, who no longer has time for them. At the other extreme, extended family members might distance themselves from the person in pain. They might feel helpless and find it easier to ignore the person than to try to figure out how to continue to have a relationship. Or they may simply want to ignore a sad situation.

Feelings of obligation and guilt often arise when one member of an extended family suffers from chronic pain. Everyone feels guilty for a different reason: the person in pain for not being who he used to be; the immediate family members for wanting to do something they enjoy despite the suffering of their loved one; and extended family members for not knowing what to do and perhaps not keeping in touch. Some families have unofficial rules of behavior for how to respond, and not everyone can comply with them. For example, in some families the expectation may be that a member visits someone who is sick on a weekly basis. This might not be possible for some members, and others may simply not want to follow this protocol. Rather than helping, such rigid, unofficial rules can make some members feel like outsiders.

Family relationships can also be strained when members yearn for the way the person in pain "used to be" rather than accepting him as he is now. The pain person may have experienced some personality changes and may be harder to communicate with because he is depressed or even angry and tyrannical. An extended family member may react by withdrawing rather than risking an argument. This can obviously influence extended family members' ability to maintain their relationships.

Extended family relationships are often more tenuous than relationships with immediate family members. As such, they are more vulnerable to rifts. Both the person in pain and her extended family must try to identify the problem and work together to resolve it. This can take time, patience, and a lot of understanding on everyone's part. It can take years for families to adjust to a new reality.

Whereas dealing with chronic pain is an entirely new situation for some families, for others it's the norm. In fact, studies show that both illness and chronic pain are subject to cultural and familial influences; this explains in part why chronic pain tends to run in families. In one study

78 percent of chronic pain patients identified at least one family member who suffered from chronic pain, compared with 44 percent in the control group. In another study, 93 percent of parents who had children with chronic pain also had extended family members with chronic pain. But just because family members have experience dealing with chronic pain doesn't mean they're particularly good at it. In fact, in many instances, just the opposite may be true: extended family members might act in ways that are not particularly useful and may even exacerbate the situation.

The story of my patient Eleanor is a good example of how one family member can negatively influence another. Eleanor came to see me complaining of severe back pain. She exhibited many chronic pain behaviors such as grimacing, groaning, and walking with a very exaggerated and stooped gait, with her hand holding her back. After examining her, I talked to Eleanor about both the physical issues surrounding her back pain and the negative influence that pain behaviors have on someone's ability to cope with chronic pain. I also mentioned that these pain behaviors usually influence other family members in a negative manner. Eleanor's eyes lit up in recognition; she told me that her husband tunes her out because she's constantly moaning and groaning. Moreover, she mentioned that her three-year-old granddaughter walks around the house holding her back and grimacing when she wants attention.

Cases like Eleanor's are not unusual. Eleanor's husband can't possibly respond to her every time she moans in pain, so he completely ignores her. By using these pain behaviors, Eleanor has effectively lost her husband's sympathy and assistance. I bet that if I were to ask Mr. Jones what was happening at home, he would tell me that he tries his best, but that he has no way of knowing when her pain is really bad and she needs help, and when her pain is tolerable and she can manage things on her own. Eleanor acts the same way all the time, and the result has been a major breakdown in communication. Of course, it's never healthy for a relationship when one spouse tunes out the other. This couple needs to learn some positive ways to cope with chronic pain.

Eleanor's pain behaviors are not only straining her marriage but also influencing other family members. Her granddaughter, who is too young to really understand the situation, is simply mimicking what she sees her grandmother do. Children, of course, mimic adults all the time—both the good things we do and the not-so-good things. Although it's impossible to tell whether Eleanor' granddaughter will grow up to have chronic pain, her home environment certainly puts her at risk.

How the Family Can Help

If someone in your family has chronic pain, there are three things you can do to help. First, establish honest and loving communication. Second, maintain a regular presence in your loved one's life. And third, find out if there are specific things you can do to make things easier for the person in pain or the immediate family. Keep in mind that adjusting to this new situation is a process, and it may take you some time to really connect with your loved one and have a positive influence in his or her life.

Communicating with someone who has chronic pain can be very difficult. Nevertheless, it's critical for family members to avoid withdrawing, even if the person in pain does not initially seem receptive. Be gently persistent about communicating. You can and should show an interest and ask questions so you understand more about what's going on. At the same time, understand that your loved one may not want to reveal certain details and that he or she has a right to privacy. It's critical that all family members respect the boundaries of other members—particularly when it comes to health issues. Choose an appropriate time and place to talk to your loved one—not during a heated argument or when the person in pain is heavily medicated or very uncomfortable. You may even want to begin the conversation by asking your loved one if she's feeling up to talking. If not, arrange another time when she's more likely to be feeling better. The best way to communicate is honestly and lovingly. You should definitely express your feelings (you have a right to feel irritated, angry, and upset), but try to do so in the kindest way possible. Keep in mind that your loved one likely feels sad and perhaps guilty about the current situation and how it impacts you and other family members.

Spending some time together on a regular basis will help with communication, send a message to your loved one that you care, and alleviate feelings of isolation. People often think they need to *do* something for someone who is ill, but frequently the best thing you can do is just check in regularly (even if it's just by phone, letters, or e-mail) so that the person in pain knows you care. Sometimes family members don't want to be around someone who's ill because it makes them feel guilty that they're healthy. Try to put things in perspective and recognize that you can best help your loved one just by being a presence in her life. At the same time, continue to enjoy your own life and do the things that bring you comfort and joy. Feeling guilty that a family member can't do what you can do doesn't help anyone. So maintain your own life and enjoy your freedom and adventures.

There are certainly things you can do to significantly help your loved one who is in pain or other family members. For example, you might provide a safe and welcome refuge for the children of someone who is ill. Consider offering to assist with errands such as grocery shopping, picking up the dry cleaning, or taking the children to school. You can cook and freeze some favorite meals, fertilize the lawn, or assist with the fall leaf cleanup. If you're handy, you can install a computer, fix a broken toilet, or put up a grab bar in the bathroom. For Christmas each year a friend of mine gives his disabled aunt the gift of his time. He goes to her house for a day to do whatever needs to be done. She makes up the list ahead of time. He arrives at a preset time and works all day doing the things she can't do for herself and would have to hire someone else to do at significant expense. If your relative can't enjoy long hikes, research accessible parks with shorter trails and places to stop and rest. At family gatherings, plan for the person's endurance and adjust the time of day and activities without making the person's condition the centerpiece. Ask your loved one what you can do to be most helpful—that way you know for sure that what you're doing is meaningful. Providing support and assistance to the spouse is also critical. For every family, the needs will be different.

Just by reading this book you have taken an important step in trying to understand more about your loved one's pain and how it affects his or her relationships. Do the best you can to maintain regular communication and contact, and ask what specific things you can do to help.

If You're the One in Pain

If you're in pain, you should have realistic expectations of what your friends and family members can do to help. You should communicate your needs and expectations directly to your loved ones; you can't expect

them to know instinctively what to do. Usually people want to help and
hesitate because they don't know how to respond. You have a right to
your privacy, but understand that isolating yourself keeps people from effectively caring for you. It's important for your family to know that you're
actively trying to reduce your pain and improve your ability to function by seeking legitimate medical treatment and following through with
your doctor's recommendations. Use words to tell people what's going
on—moans and groans will only alienate them. Although being honest
and sharing your feelings is important, being overly critical or constantly
complaining will just drive people away. If family members offer to help,
suggest concrete ways they can assist. If there's really nothing they can
do, then let them know that just caring about you and expressing concern is enough. If you have family members who are avoiding or ignoring you, try to be the first one to reach out. Chances are they just don't
know what to do.

We can't assume that people who want to help will intuitively know
what to do. As many new mothers can attest, often those who are most
willing to lend a hand don't know how best to do so. For example, after I
gave birth to each of my children, a number of lovely people wanted to
pitch in. Unfortunately, in the beginning the offer to help consisted of a
friend or family member holding my newborn while I did whatever
needed to be done around the house. Not feeling physically up to doing
chores, I often just sat and talked to them while they held my newborn—
something I would rather have been doing. With each child I got a little
bit better at communicating what people could really do to help (for example, folding laundry or picking up diapers at the store), and their assistance was a wonderful relief.

Although asking for help is important, at the same time you need to
stay as independent as possible. You should continue to do everything
you can to care for yourself and your immediate family. It's sometimes
easy to start letting others take over, and it can be a subtle process that
you might not easily recognize until you find yourself more disabled
than you really need to be. You may be in that situation now—where
even *you* don't recognize your potential because it's become so hidden by
the efforts of others. Try to strike a balance between letting people assist
you and continuing to remain as independent as possible. If you don't
need or want help at all, then invite your loved one simply to visit with

you or take an outing together. Take the time to enjoy the things you still can and share them with the important people in your life.

It's absolutely essential for people who live with chronic pain to address not only the physical pain but also the psychological effects of the illness. When you find yourself caught in a cycle of low self-esteem and hopelessness, focus on what you like best about yourself. Ask yourself what contribution you can make to your family, your neighborhood, or your community. What can you do to make others happy? Is there something you don't like about yourself that you have the power to change? What do you do that makes you feel good?

Positive self-esteem goes hand in hand with maintaining a sense of hope. Cheri Register speaks and writes about chronic illness after having lived with Caroli's disease, a rare and painful inherited disorder of the liver. In her book *The Chronic Illness Experience*, she writes, "How well people manage lives marked by chronic illness depends not on the nature of the illness but on the strength of their conviction that life is worth living no matter what complications are imposed on it."[1] It's important for you to feel as though your life has purpose *despite the pain*. If you're feeling sad or even hopeless, try to recognize these feelings. One way to maintain hope is to set some personal goals. For example, consider taking correspondence courses to finish a postponed degree, or take a course on art, music, or dance for enjoyment. Consider volunteering time to a favorite cause or making something for an annual fundraiser.

When I counsel patients, I tell them to think of their energy as money. You only have so much; how do you want to spend it? What's meaningful to you? Keep in mind that everything can't be a top priority; you have to pick and choose, as we all do, what you want to accomplish in your life. For example, I usually save time and energy by ordering my groceries online and having them delivered. Some of my patients balk when I suggest that they do this, because they're gourmet cooks who thoroughly enjoy shopping for the finest foods and then cooking delicious meals for their families. Another one of my patients is a Jehovah's Witness who wants to spend her time going door to door talking to people about her faith. What's important to one person is not necessarily of consequence to others, so think about what matters most to you and pursue it— whether it's cooking a gourmet meal, talking to people about your religion, volunteering at your local food pantry, or coaching your child's soccer team. Determine what your priorities are, start small, and build on your success. If your negative feelings persist or you're actively depressed, seek help from a mental health professional. Depression is a treatable condition, and if left untreated it will only add to your health problems. Moreover, your emotional well being affects everyone around you. One of the best things you can do for yourself and your family is to improve your psychological state.

Although living with chronic pain may drastically change your life, you can take some positive steps to improve your relationships with loved ones. Work on establishing and maintaining regular communication with extended family members. Avoid being overly critical or complaining incessantly. Let them share some positive experiences with you —even if it's just a pleasant game of cards or an engaging chat. Remain as active as possible, but if you need help give people specific suggestions and keep them from guessing what they should do. Finally, if you are feeling sad or depressed, seek professional help. You may have no choice about living with pain, but you can improve your emotional well being.

9

Emotional Changes and Depression

JEFF grew up with an alcoholic father who beat him regularly. As an adult he became completely dysfunctional and relied on heroin to get through the day. A junkie who spent twenty years on the streets, he supported his drug habit through prostitution, stealing, and anything else that netted him a quick dollar. When he wasn't on the streets he was in jail. He finally kicked his habit and went back to school. He has finished his bachelor's degree and master's degree and is now working on his doctorate. Jeff appears to be much older than his forty-five years. Years of hard living have taken their toll—he is overweight, balding, and missing several teeth. Sleeping on hard surfaces and several motorcycle accidents have left Jeff with multiple injuries and chronic neck and back pain. Yet every time I see him he's smiling, and he always tells me that things are going well. One day I asked him how he did it—how he quit using drugs and began to face both the emotional and the physical pain. Jeff told me that for years he was angry and depressed. He felt cheated in having such a terrible life, and he blamed his father for starting a vicious cycle of physical and emotional pain. Jeff gradually decided that he had the power to change his situation. He entered a drug rehabilitation program and began seeing a psychiatrist regularly. He started taking medications that helped with both his depression and his physical pain. Then he went back to school so that he could become a counselor and someday help other people.

Jeff's is ultimately a success story, but during the years that he was depressed and on drugs, he married four women and had eight children. He abandoned them all, and only recently has he established contact with two of his children—the others won't have anything to do with him.

Jeff is about to marry wife number five. For the first time in his life, he plans to start a family when he's clean and sober and working a legitimate job. Jeff's antidote to his chronic pain and depression is hard work and a dedication to having a better life. Although in the past he has been destructive to himself and to his family, he is now an honorable man who plans to be a devoted husband and father.

Jeff's case is fairly extreme, but studies reveal that more than 50 percent of people with chronic pain suffer from depression. Other emotions such as anxiety, grief, loss, shame, denial, guilt, fear, and anger are also quite prevalent. Research shows that many people with chronic pain come from abusive backgrounds. A history of childhood physical abuse is equally common in men and women who suffer from chronic pain, and among women pain sufferers there are also increased rates of sexual abuse and domestic violence. Moreover, people who have both pain and depression are at a greater risk of unemployment and a dysfunctional family life. This is true regardless of ethnic background, gender, or age.

Emotional changes, particularly depression, are influenced by a variety of factors. In pain medicine, these are commonly referred to as *biopsychosocial* influences. The biopsychosocial model for the treatment of chronic pain is based on the importance of addressing not only the biological factors (for example, heredity and chemical reactions in the brain) but also psychological factors (such as anxiety, depression, perceived control over pain, and so on) and social factors (for example, family and work environment). These three categories sometimes overlap, but they provide us with an important basis for exploring what causes pain and depression.

Biological Factors

There are many chemical reactions that occur in the brain, and some of these greatly impact mood and pain levels. Two compounds, serotonin and noradrenaline, have an influence on *both* depression and pain. Though it is not entirely clear how the compounds are related, evidence points to a definite link. Functional imaging of the brain (such as positron emission tomography, known as PET scans, and functional magnetic resonance imaging, or MRI scans) is becoming increasingly important in researching how the brain reacts with respect to both pain and depression. For example, in a functional imaging study we can assess what happens to cerebral blood flow when a painful stimulus is given. Gene therapy is also providing a wealth of information on the biology of pain and mood disorders. We know that there are relationships between the two, but at this time they're still not well understood.

Medications used to treat pain can sometimes be identical to drugs used to treat depression, a further indication that the two conditions are somehow related. But some medications that are used to treat pain may actually *worsen* symptoms of fatigue and depression, so doctors must consider both conditions when prescribing drugs that alter the brain's chemical balance. Other biological factors in the development of chronic pain include a family history of chronic pain, depression, or both. Someone with a prior history of depression is more likely to become depressed again if he develops a chronic pain condition. We also know that people who have a history of depression are more likely to develop chronic pain than those who have no prior depression. It's possible that in this subset of patients there's a genetic predisposition to both conditions. Children of parents in pain may become depressed owing to a genetic predisposition (which is a biological factor) and/or the fact that they may not have good coping skills (a social factor).

Psychological Factors

Genetic predisposition to emotional imbalances aside, we know that psychological factors play a significant role in chronic pain, and that both depression and anxiety often *precede* the pain. Most people who complain of pain have real physical pain, but occasionally people who are depressed will complain of pain without really experiencing significant discomfort. They don't do this intentionally to deceive anyone—some people just believe that pain is a more acceptable medical problem than depression. Usually these patients don't even realize that their main problem is a psychological one. Mental health professionals call this type of chronic pain a "depressive equivalent," which means that the real problem is depression, not pain.

Physicians treating people who have chronic pain and depression (or anxiety) must consider psychological factors. For example, the fear of further injury may cause someone with a pain condition to curtail activities that she's perfectly capable of doing, which can lead to a "learned helplessness." This can also lead to a diminished sense of self-worth and social isolation. It's important to correct a common (and mistaken) assumption about the *severity* of pain: often people believe that the severity of their pain symptoms indicates the severity of their illness—so if they're in severe pain, they're anxious and fearful because they assume that their illness must be very bad. This does not hold true with chronic pain—very severe pain does not necessarily mean that the prognosis is dire or that the condition is worsening. One of my colleagues who is a pain doctor describes chronic pain (in most instances) to his patients as "safe pain," meaning that the severity of the pain (that is, whether you're having a "good day" or a "bad day") does not reflect the severity or progression of the illness. He reassures patients that when they have pain it's still safe to do the things they enjoy. Of course, this is a generalization, and though it holds true for most chronic pain conditions, you should always discuss with your own physician the limitations of your particular condition.

Naturally, people in pain and their families experience worry and distress, and these emotions don't necessarily lead to full-blown anxiety or depression. But they sometimes can in susceptible individuals. It's important for people with chronic pain and their loved ones to recognize that there's a relationship between how well someone functions emotionally and how well they can manage their pain and their day-to-day life. If you or someone in your family begins to experience more severe symptoms of anxiety or depression, consult a professional who has experience with mental health issues.

Individuals with chronic pain tend to have more suicidal thoughts and attempts than the general population. Chronic medical illness has been identified as a motivating factor in as many as 25 percent of suicides, with less than 4 percent occurring in the context of a terminal illness. In one published survey, 50 percent of people with chronic pain reported that they had at some point seriously considered suicide. Suicide is also more frequent in people who are depressed and in those who abuse alcohol. A history of previous attempts is also a risk factor for suicide.

One day a patient at the center where I work began having flashbacks about his accident, an electrocution injury that left him partially paralyzed and with severe intractable pain. He became agitated and the center staff summoned me to handle the emergency (his treating physician was not on site). By the time I arrived, the patient had become suicidal. As my staff called 911, I told the patient that we needed to make sure he didn't hurt himself. He needed to go to the hospital, where he could be assessed by a psychiatrist who would determine when it was safe for him to return home to his wife and children. The patient readily agreed to go by ambulance. Unfortunately, his story is not unique—every pain doctor is acutely aware of the risk of suicide in patients who are experiencing both chronic pain and emotional instability. People in pain and their families should also be aware of this issue and seek professional help immediately if there's any indication at all that someone is considering suicide as an option, whether or not the threat seems serious.

Social Factors

Family, friends, and colleagues all play a significant role in how someone copes with the physical and emotional consequences of chronic pain. People who have strong social support systems tend to cope better, with fewer emotional problems, than those who do not have a lot of support. Anyone who becomes severely depressed, whether that person began with a good support system or not, can become socially isolated owing to the emotional illness and how he or she copes with it. Even the most loving spouse might feel like giving up if a partner who is in pain and depressed is uncommunicative, sad, and angry. Moreover, even individuals who have a great home life can become depressed if they're out of work, in litigation, or unable to pursue the interests that give life variety and meaning.

What the Person in Pain Can Do

If you're in pain and struggling emotionally, there are a number of things you can do to help yourself. First, admit and accept your loss. It's essential for you to understand that pain feeds depression and depression feeds pain. The same is true for anxiety and other mood disturbances. Although this may seem like a vicious cycle, you can break the cycle by first recognizing it and then taking responsibility for your treatment—both physically and psychologically.

Once you've overcome the first hurdle, you're ready to seek assistance.

There are many professionals who can help. You may need to consult a mental health professional who specializes in treating anxiety and depression in the context of illness and chronic pain. Although some psychiatrists continue to counsel patients, the current trend in medicine is for them to focus on starting and adjusting medications that help treat symptoms of anxiety and depression. Psychologists and clinical social workers, who are not licensed to prescribe medications, perform counseling. Because emotional issues play such an important part in chronic pain conditions, many chronic pain treatment programs offer mental health counseling in addition to other pain services. Your primary care physician should also be able to recommend a qualified mental health professional with expertise in chronic pain.

While some patients will need long-term psychotherapy to address complicated issues such as substance abuse, a history of childhood abuse, or post-traumatic stress disorder that may have resulted from a serious injury, as was the case with the gentleman described earlier who was electrocuted, many people with chronic pain will simply need a few counseling sessions to complete short-term goals. These goals can include making a realistic plan to change their circumstances as well as to learn cognitive strategies to help reduce stress and anxiety (for example, biofeedback or imagery). The counselor should also be able to provide accurate information about a particular medical condition in order to eliminate unrealistic fears.

Medications are an important consideration in the treatment of emotional issues. Since depression and anxiety are typically due to chemical imbalances in the brain, your doctor might suggest medications that will help improve your mood. Your doctor should also take the time to review your current medications to be sure that none of them is contributing to mood disturbances. This is a common problem that can be improved with proper dosing or elimination of the offending drug. You should avoid self-medicating with alcohol or other substances. Alcohol is a depressant, and though people sometimes use it to help lessen feelings of anxiety and frustration, it almost always has the opposite effect, particularly when used regularly.

Trusted friends, family members, or clergy can be good listeners. It's important to share your feelings with someone you trust. Communicating with your loved ones is an essential part of improving your psychological health, and it's also an important part of maintaining good relationships with people who support you. Some people will also benefit from joining a support group consisting of others who are suffering with the same or a similar illness. Keeping a journal can also be a safe way to let your feelings out.

Once you've admitted your loss and are seeking help, the final thing you have to do is find ways to boost your self-esteem and to challenge yourself. In his book *How Good Do We Have to Be?* Rabbi Kushner writes, "There is a wholeness about the person who has come to terms with his limitations, who knows who he is and what he can and cannot do, the person who has been brave enough to let go of his unrealistic dreams and not feel like a failure for doing so."[1] One way to challenge yourself is by becoming more physically active. Exercise releases chemicals in the brain that have a positive effect on mood. Moreover, exercise is a good way to improve your overall health, and if done properly (check with your doctor on this) it might help to reduce your pain level. There are many

Symptoms of Depression

Loss of interest in usual activities and pastimes
Irritability
Frequent crying
Sadness
Hopelessness
Poor appetite or significant weight loss
Increased appetite or significant weight gain
Sleeping poorly
Sleeping too much
Agitation or restlessness
Fatigue (particularly in the morning after a night's rest)
Difficulty concentrating
Difficulty making decisions
Feeling self-critical
Excessive guilt
Feelings of worthlessness
Recurrent thoughts of dying or suicidal thoughts

(continued)

Symptoms of Anxiety

Feeling tense or nervous
Feeling jittery or jumpy
Difficulty relaxing
Fatigue
Muscle aches
Restlessness
Apprehension
Fearfulness or anticipation of misfortune
Feeling sweaty or having clammy hands
Chest palpitations or racing heart
Stomachache
Lightheadedness or dizziness
Difficulty sleeping
Feeling "on edge"
Feeling terrified without apparent reason
Anticipation of impending doom
Shortness of breath
Choking or smothering sensation
Feeling faint
Trembling or shaking

other ways to boost your self-esteem and challenge yourself—if you need specific suggestions, ask the people you trust to help.

What the Family Can Do

The patient must do most of the work involved in treating chronic pain and any emotional issues that stem from it. Families can be supportive and can certainly have a positive influence, but the person in pain must be the one to seek help and follow through with treatment. As a family member, you can help by recognizing whether your loved one is experiencing emotional issues that need to be addressed by a mental health professional. If you think the person in pain needs professional help, encourage him in this direction. You might offer to go to the appointment and lend support. Often people who are depressed can't concentrate very well, so if the person in pain is amenable, you can help him by writing out questions to ask the doctor.

Family members should also recognize self-destructive behavior, or behavior that harms other people in the family, especially children. It's extremely important for you to intervene and seek appropriate professional help if your loved one is in any way abusive to others. It's also critical to intervene if your loved one voices any thoughts about hurting him- or herself. Watch out for prescription medication abuse, alcohol abuse, and illicit drug abuse as well. Many chronic pain treatment programs involve the family, so this would be a good time to bring up these issues. Another option is to talk to your loved one's doctor about your concerns. Most doctors will listen to what family members have to say but won't give them any information about the patient without the patient's consent. When family members approach me with their concerns, I always tell them, "You can tell me anything you want, but I can't reveal anything to you without your loved one's consent."

Although psychological issues can be as disabling or even more disabling than the physical pain, there is almost always help for individuals who are experiencing emotional problems. Gerald Sittser, who lost his mother, wife, and four-year-old daughter in a terrible car accident, writes in his memoir, *A Grace Disguised,* "The decision to face the darkness, even if it led to overwhelming pain, showed me that the experience of loss itself does not have to be the defining moment of our lives. Instead, the defining moment can be *our response* to the loss."[2]

10

Medication Dependence and Addiction

A FEW years ago one of my patients, a lawyer with chronic neck and arm pain, came in very disgruntled because I had written in a medical note that I was concerned about placing him on long-term narcotics owing to the risk of addiction. He felt that he was the type of person who would never become addicted to anything, and he also thought that my statement might be a red flag to a life or disability insurer. He had some good points, but he was also generally misinformed about the risks associated with long-term use of opioid painkillers. Although there are several classes of medications that can be abused, the most common ones are pain relievers, sedatives and tranquilizers, and stimulants. According to the National Survey on Drug Use and Health (NSDUH), a project of the Substance Abuse and Mental Health Services Administration (SAMHSA), in 2002 an estimated 6.2 million people were using prescription medications for nonmedical purposes.[1] Of these, 4.4 million were misusing pain relievers. Older people may be at greatest risk for misuse because they have a higher incidence of painful medical conditions and are prescribed medications about three times as frequently as the general population.

It's important to begin with an understanding of narcotics, which are now usually called *opioid analgesics*. Opium is a naturally occurring substance that comes from poppy juice. It contains a number of chemicals such as morphine and codeine. Some opioids are also synthetically made in the laboratory. These potent painkillers, whether they occur naturally or are synthetically produced, attach to specific proteins called opioid receptors (which are found in the brain, spinal cord, and gastrointestinal tract) and block the transmission of pain messages to the brain. They

Side Effects of Opioids

Rash/itching
Nausea/vomiting
Constipation
Sedation
Dizziness
Cognitive impairment
Respiratory depression
Urinary retention

have the potential to cause drug *tolerance, physical dependence, addiction,* and *abuse.* These conditions should not be confused with *side effects,* which are potential negative physical reactions that can occur with all medications. Serious side effects of opioids can include respiratory depression (slowed breathing), so it's recommended that these medications not be used in conjunction with alcohol, antihistamines, barbiturates, or benzodiazepines. It's important to note that the nomenclature used to describe opioid-related effects is not completely standardized, and the terms are often used incorrectly. In order to have a useful discussion, however, I will define the terms initially and use the commonly accepted definitions. Note that I use the terms "medications" and "drugs" interchangeably to mean prescription medications. When I address other substances, I will explicitly state what I'm referring to.

The use of opioids to treat chronic pain is a hotly debated issue. There is little disagreement among the experts about the benefits of these medications for people with terminal diseases such as cancer. But for people of all ages who do not have end-stage cancer, there is decided controversy about whether these drugs should be prescribed. This is not the place to enter into the debate—it's a difficult issue with compelling arguments on both sides. Instead, I'll present the problems associated with medications that have the potential for physical dependence and addiction.

Because many prescription medications can result in problems with patient tolerance, physical dependence, addiction, and abuse, the United States Drug Enforcement Agency (DEA) supervises these so-called

U.S. DEA Classification for Scheduled Substances

Schedule I   No accepted medical use (for example, street drugs such
                as heroin and LSD)

Schedule II   High addiction potential with severe dependence liability
                (for example, morphine, oxycodone, amphetamines,
                secobarbital)

Schedule III   Less addiction potential than schedules I and II (for
                example, acetaminophen that contains limited
                quantities of certain narcotics, such as Tylenol with
                codeine)

Schedule IV   Less addiction potential than schedules I–III (for
                example, phenobarbital, benzodiazepines,
                propoxyphene, pentazocine, phentermine)

Schedule V   Least addiction potential of scheduled substances (for
                example, buprenorphine, propylhexedrine)

scheduled substances. Often called *controlled substances,* many of these drugs have a "street value" and are sold illegally on the black market. Drugs in these classes are supervised by the DEA, and physicians are required to fill out a special application and to use a DEA number in order to prescribe them. Although there are many scheduled drugs, much of the discussion in this chapter focuses on opioids (narcotics), since most of the research has been done on this class of medications and because they most commonly prove problematic with chronic pain patients.

Tolerance

Tolerance occurs when someone requires an increased dose of medication to experience the same level of pain relief (that is, after many doses, the drug becomes less effective in managing pain). Tolerance to opioids often occurs early in the course of treatment. If a patient requires ever higher doses of medication, the doctor must consider whether the pain is worsening or the individual is becoming addicted to the drug. The prescribing physician must carefully assess anyone who requires increasing doses of any scheduled substance. Another potential problem with

Signs of Opioid Withdrawal versus Intoxication

WITHDRAWAL

Increase in saliva and tears

Yawning

Enlarged pupils

Gooseflesh

Tremors

Inability to sleep

Decreased appetite

Vomiting

Diarrhea

Irritability

Increased blood pressure

Muscle cramps

Drug craving

Bad mood

INTOXICATION

Insensitivity to pain

Drowsiness

Euphoria

Mental clouding

Constricted pupils

Vomiting

Difficulty breathing

opioids is "cross-tolerance," which means that repeated exposure to an opioid may result in tolerance not only to the drug being used but also to other opioids.

Physical Dependence

Physical dependence occurs after more than just a few days of continuous use and results in symptoms of withdrawal when the medication is abruptly discontinued. Physical dependence is usually not a problem as long as patients are told to wean themselves off these medications rather

Criteria for Diagnosing Prescription Drug Addiction

1. Patient exhibits tolerance.
2. Withdrawal symptoms expected to occur if drug is stopped abruptly (physical dependence).
3. Substance is taken in larger amounts and/or over a longer period of time than was intended.
4. Patient is unsuccessful at reducing and controlling the medication.
5. Much time is spent trying to obtain the medication.
6. Important social, occupational, or recreational activities are given up or reduced because of medication use.
7. Drug is continued despite knowledge that it likely caused or exacerbated a physical or psychological problem.

than stopping them abruptly. Drug dependence and tolerance both describe *physical* problems and *do not* indicate either addiction or abuse. But it's important to note that both tolerance and physical dependence are part of the criteria for diagnosing a substance addiction problem.

Many of my patients have not appreciated the power of their medication to induce physical dependence. Fred, an executive at a well-known company, began using a combination of Valium and Percocet after a car accident left him with severe neck pain and chronic headaches. Fred was referred to me by his primary care physician, who did not think that Fred's neurologist was helping him by continuously prescribing these medications. In fact, when I talked to Fred, he told me that the medications didn't seem to be helping him, and he admitted that he didn't feel as mentally sharp as he needed to be in his business. We agreed that he would wean off these medications and try some other, non-pharmacologic treatments including physical therapy, acupuncture, and massage. At the next visit, Fred said that he felt much better off the medications, "but I went through hell when I stopped them." Fred had decided to ignore my advice about carefully tapering the medications so as to avoid symptoms of withdrawal and instead decided to stop them abruptly (a potentially dangerous move). He didn't believe that his body had become physically dependent on them, and he had been eager to try another treatment approach. Because many patients don't appreciate how serious withdrawal symptoms can be, I spend a lot of time in my office emphasizing the fact that they need to slowly taper medications that have the potential to induce physical dependence.

Addiction

Addiction in general is characterized by compulsive use and craving of any substance that is used for mood-altering purposes. Individuals are addicted to an opioid (or any other drug) if they (1) lose control over the use of the medication; (2) compulsively use the medication; (3) crave the medication; and (4) continue to use the medication despite the possibility of harm to themselves or others. The American Society of Addiction

Appropriate Medication Use versus Addiction

PAIN PATIENT WHO USES MEDICATIONS APPROPRIATELY

- Uses the medication as prescribed.
- Experiences improvement in function and physical abilities on the medication.
- Displays an awareness of and concern with the issues in chronic opioid use.
- Follows agreed-upon treatment plan and does not rely exclusively on narcotics.
- Has medications left over from previous prescriptions.

ADDICTED PAIN PATIENT

- Uses the medication more often than prescribed.
- Does not experience improved function or physical abilities on the drug.
- Continues to complain of intolerable pain and requests more medication without appropriate concern.
- Does not comply with treatment plan.
- Runs out of the prescription early or loses prescription—always has a "story."

Medicine considers addiction "a disease process characterized by the continued use of a specific psychoactive substance despite physical, psychological, or social harm." In other words, addiction is a medical condition that manifests as a psychological and behavioral problem.

Addiction occurs in up to 20 percent of individuals who use opioids for chronic pain and is more common in people with a past history of substance addiction, family history of addiction, or prior psychiatric problems (for example, depression and anxiety). Many people who are susceptible to addiction become addicted to more than one medication and may abuse street drugs and alcohol at the same time that they're improperly taking medications. In some instances, people with chronic pain will not become addicted to prescription drugs but will self-medicate with alcohol or illicit drugs to try to control the pain. These substances have mood-altering properties and can be highly addictive, which helps explain why many individuals with chronic pain who become addicted have great difficulty functioning at work, socially, and at home. They might use medications in dangerous situations such as while driving a car or operating machinery; and they might even run afoul of the law (facing arrest for falsifying prescriptions or for disorderly conduct). Moreover, people who are addicted continue to use the offending medication despite serious disruptions to personal and professional life (for example, absences from work, tardiness with work deadlines, arguments with spouse and children, and so on) that are caused by or exacerbated by the effects of the substance.

Families are thrown into turmoil when a loved one becomes addicted to medications. In many instances, family members think that the person in pain is the one with the problem, but addiction affects the entire family. Family members often become frustrated and angry at all the broken promises the person in pain is unable to fulfill (for example, pledges to reduce or eliminate the medication or avoid missing work). They're often ashamed of their loved one and sometimes go to great lengths to keep others from learning about their "dirty little secret." In his book *Prescription Drug Addiction: The Hidden Epidemic*, author Rod Colvin, who lost his brother to an overdose of prescription medications mixed with alcohol, describes two levels of "enabling"—the innocent phase and the desperate phase.[2] In the innocent phase, family members help to protect the person in pain because they think that she's just going through a "rough period." An example of this kind of enabling would be calling an employer and saying that the person in pain can't come to work because she's sick (rather than incapacitated by medication) or paying for a traffic ticket rather than confronting the person in pain over the true cause of the violation. In the desperate phase, the family realizes that the person in pain is addicted, but they're so worried about the consequences (loss of employment, jail time) that they actually step up the enabling process to further protect her. In this phase the family may do things like pay rent or medical expenses rather than address the addiction problem.

People with chronic pain are often in denial about the fact that they're addicted, and this denial has enormous consequences for how the family functions. Family members may complain to the person in pain about his behavior, lack of follow through, and irresponsibility. They may confront him about the addiction problem, which can lead to heated arguments or other relationship problems. Alternatively, family members might be in denial themselves. They may not want to admit that their loved one has a problem with addiction, or they may feel that their relative is entitled to use the medication to treat pain regardless of the problems associated with it. Whatever the case, understand that addiction is a *progressive medical condition that worsens without treatment.*

Abuse

Abuse occurs when someone uses a substance in a way that deviates from approved medical use or social patterns within society. Abuse conveys cultural disapproval and is often associated with the "recreational" use of substances. Approximately one-third of the U.S. population has used illicit drugs. An estimated 6–15 percent of the population has some form of substance-use disorder. People are most familiar with abuse in the context of illegal street drugs; however, it's estimated that up to 28 percent of controlled substances are abused. Moreover, it's estimated that more than four million Americans use prescription drugs for nonmedical purposes. Prescription medications are often "diverted" from legitimate channels to illicit ones via falsified prescriptions.

Another way people who are addicted get large quantities of controlled substances is to "doctor shop." Many patients go from doctor to doctor asking for the same or similar medications. In the past, doctors had no

way of knowing what other physicians had prescribed for someone; however, with modern technology we often have easy access to this information. For example, Marty was sent to me by his primary care physician for
low back pain. His doctor told me on the phone that he thought Marty
needed some strong pain medications, but that he didn't want to prescribe them. I saw Marty once and gave him a prescription for a few narcotic pills. A few days later he called and said that his pills had disappeared when his luggage was lost. I immediately suspected a problem
and called his pharmacy. The pharmacist said that my prescription was
the only controlled substance on record for Marty. I then called his health
insurer, who informed me that Marty had filled prescriptions for narcotics at twenty different pharmacies over the past three months. I confronted Marty with what I had discovered, and not surprisingly, he de-
nied everything and told me that his insurer must be confusing him with
someone else. I then called the airline (with Marty in the room), and they
told me they had no record of Marty's flying with them recently and no
record of losing his luggage. Marty repeatedly made up excuses as I
counseled him to get help. He left my office and never came back. I later
heard that both Marty and his wife were addicted to opioids and that
Marty was the one who would "doctor shop" for both of them.

Avoiding Addiction

When prescribing opioid analgesia for chronic pain, physicians can do a
number of things to minimize the risk of addiction. It goes without saying that they should be knowledgeable about the risks associated with all
the medications they prescribe. Furthermore, they need to inform patients about both the benefits and the risks associated with the medications they prescribe. Most doctors are aware that potent and high-dose
opioids can and should be liberally prescribed in cases of severe acute
pain (for example, after surgery) or in instances where someone has a
terminal cancer that's very painful. In these types of situations there are
relatively few, if any, addiction issues to address. This is because individuals with severe, acute pain do *not* become addicted to medications with
short-term use. Addiction becomes an issue only when patients use certain medications for a prolonged period of time—such as in chronic
pain. It's hard to tell how long it will take someone to become addicted,

Sample Opioid Treatment Contract

I, [PATIENT'S NAME], AGREE TO THE FOLLOWING CONDITIONS:

1. I understand that I have a chronic pain problem that will be treated with opioid medications in order to increase my function. The risks and benefits of this medication have been fully explained to me.

2. I will obtain prescriptions for opioids only from [doctor's name].

3. I will have my prescriptions filled only at [pharmacy name and address].

4. I will take my medication only as prescribed.

5. I agree to random urine and blood tests to assess my compliance.

6. I will keep all scheduled appointments with [doctor's name].

7. I understand that lost, misplaced, or stolen medications will not be replaced.

8. I understand that if I deviate from these stated guidelines or the medication loses its effectiveness in increasing my function, it will be promptly tapered and discontinued.

Signature of patient_____Date_____

but the risk is exceedingly low in the first couple of weeks of treatment. On the other hand, both physical tolerance and side effects can develop quickly, so it's a good rule of thumb for doctors to wean all controlled substances and monitor patients throughout their treatment for evidence of side effects.

Certain individuals with chronic pain are more susceptible to addictive tendencies than others, and the treating physician should assess patients for these risk factors. They include a prior history of prescription medication addiction, past history of illicit drug use, or family history of addiction to any substance. Doctors should also assess whether someone is psychologically stable and has consistently followed through with past treatment recommendations in a responsible manner. Although opioids are not contraindicated in someone with severe anxiety or depression, it's important that the individual be emotionally stable enough to take the medications as prescribed.

Weak versus Strong Opioids

WEAK OPIOIDS

Codeine

Dextropropoxyphene

Dihydrocodeine

STRONG OPIOIDS

Buprenorphine

Methadone

Morphine

Oxycodone

Pentazocine

Doctors who prescribe opioids in chronic pain patients should ideally follow these guidelines: (1) have an established relationship with the patient; (2) begin treatment with a trial that has defined goals (often doctors will ask their patients to sign a formal contract that outlines those goals); (3) continue medication only if side effects are controlled and the patient demonstrates clear benefit through improved function; (4) start the trial with a weak opioid at a low dose and increase as needed; (5) if continuous pain relief is required, avoid short-acting medications that are given on an as-needed basis (long-acting opiates that are taken regularly are usually a better option); (6) consider combining medications rather than just using a single drug; (7) prescribe opioids in combination with other non-pharmacologic pain treatments (for example, physical therapy or acupuncture); (8) monitor patients carefully and frequently.

If you're suffering from chronic pain, you can do a lot to minimize your risk of addiction to prescription medications by ensuring that you're well informed about the drugs you're taking and by investigating other (both pharmacologic and non-pharmacologic) treatment options. In addition, you should follow your doctor's recommendations regarding dosing and be sure to keep all follow-up appointments. If you start to feel out of control with respect to medication use, discuss your concerns with your doctor as soon as possible. While "being in denial" has become a catchphrase in our culture, it remains a dangerous reality of addiction. Pay careful attention to what your friends and family members are telling you if they notice problems involving your medication use.

Confronting and Overcoming Addiction

Treating someone who has both chronic pain and a prescription medication addiction is always a challenge. Once someone becomes addicted to one drug, future pain-control options become much more limited. Addiction can be more debilitating than chronic pain, however, so it's important to put the problem into perspective. In almost all instances, overcoming addiction means giving up the offending medication and usually most other drugs that could potentially be abused. Although complete detoxification (that is, giving up all medications with abuse potential) is usually the preferred method of handling addictions, there are some alternatives, including methadone maintenance (methadone has been found to be an effective way of controlling some people's substance addiction and abuse problems) or regular attendance at a very strict chronic pain clinic where the medication doses are carefully monitored and medication use is scrutinized to prevent opportunities for abuse. Both of these options are very time-consuming and typically work for a minority of patients. Most people who become addicted to prescription medications need to undergo complete detoxification under professional guidance at a short-term hospital based at a residential drug-treatment facility.

Once you recognize that you have a problem, the next step is to seek help. You can call Narcotics Anonymous, or, if you have a doctor you can trust, talk to him or her about your concerns. In order to deal effectively with addiction, you'll need to have a plan that makes sense medically. Abruptly discontinuing a medication can be dangerous, and you may need alternative pain-control options. If you don't have a doctor in whom you can confide then consult a therapist, if possible. Clinical social workers and psychologists typically have a lot of experience in helping people with addiction issues. If you can't confide in a doctor or a therapist, then find someone you can trust (a family member, friend, or clergy).

Many people successfully conquer addictions through twelve-step support groups such as Narcotics Anonymous. Asking for help is a critical first step.

Detoxing is an essential part of dealing with your addiction. You can do this at home, but it can be dangerous. You might feel isolated, depressed, anxious, fearful, or confused. Going through withdrawal alone and without guidance is not advisable. There are formal treatment programs dedicated to addiction, and if at all possible, you should try to join one of them. They can be inpatient- or outpatient-based. The advantages of a treatment facility include medication management, support groups, a safe environment, supervised detoxification, suicide watch, and monitoring of vital signs. Moreover, the environment is usually nonjudgmental and the emphasis is on decreasing loneliness and isolation and encouraging healthy lifestyle changes. Addiction treatment programs often offer family counseling and participation that can be crucial to helping you maintain your sobriety. Although the term "enabling" has become a cliché, family members' behaviors can often unwittingly contribute to a loved one's substance abuse problem. It's just as essential for family members to learn well behaviors as it is for you to learn them. Moreover, understand that it's not uncommon for someone to detox and then say, "Now that I'm off mind-altering substances, I can see that I don't have a life." The support of your family and friends, even if you have alienated them while you were addicted, can be enormously beneficial to you once you're off the toxic medications. Professional guidance for both you and your family is essential.

Once you have completed the detoxification process, you will need to have follow-up support from professionals. Nearly everyone in this situation will benefit from having a therapist to talk to, as this is usually a very difficult transition time and one in which many people will relapse. In order to have a successful recovery, you should at least have a pain doctor who can help you manage the pain without medications that are potentially addictive, and a therapist who understands addiction and can continue to reinforce your recovery. You may also need to see a psychiatrist if you're experiencing psychological issues such as depression and anxiety.

If you have a loved one who is addicted, then the entire family is probably suffering. Help is available; a number of organizations will provide information and assistance to families and individuals in crisis (see Appendix). If you've already tried having a one-on-one talk with your loved one and it didn't work, consider an intervention. Interventions can take many different forms and can involve a variety of people. The purpose of an intervention is to break through the addicted person's denial and excuses for not seeking treatment and to get her to either commit to treatment or immediately enter a treatment facility (which means that at the conclusion of the intervention, the individual is driven directly to a facility that is waiting to accept her). Family members are usually an integral part of an intervention, though friends can sometimes be involved as well. Often it's useful to have a therapist present to help facilitate or to lead the intervention.

Interventions are most successful when the addicted individual is confronted in a loving and supportive manner. Members of the intervention "team" should be prepared for the addicted person to come up with excuses such as "I can't miss time from work." Rehearsing responses to the issues that will likely be raised can greatly improve the chances of success (for example, telling your loved one, "You have sick leave and it's time to start taking care of yourself"). If you're unable to convince your loved one to seek treatment, you have few options. This doesn't mean that you should give up, but recognize that you cannot control someone else's behavior. Information and support are available for family members trying to cope with this difficult issue. By understanding addiction and seeking different solutions that have worked for others, you can do a lot to help not only your loved one who is addicted but also your entire family. But bear in mind that no matter what you do, ultimately your loved one must admit the problem in order to get help.

11

Diagnosing Chronic Pain Conditions

A COUPLE of years ago Margaret, a woman in her early forties, came to see me for chronic hip pain. Margaret reported that she had been to several doctors and that after three years I was her "last hope." She described severe, disabling pain along the sides of her thighs. The pain was so intense that she was unable to play sports with her young son and even found it difficult to walk at times. She had stopped going to malls and had curtailed most activities that involved walking for more than a few feet. Her world had shrunk to the point where she just did the bare necessities—going to work, grocery shopping, and picking her son up at school. She was miserable and had little hope of feeling better after all this time.

As Margaret relayed her story, I was curious to know how other doctors had diagnosed and treated her. She told me that her primary care doctor had diagnosed "hip arthritis" and treated her with anti-inflammatory medications. When that didn't help, she went to see a specialist in rheumatology who confirmed the diagnosis of hip arthritis and gave her a different anti-inflammatory medication. He also told Margaret that she may need to consider a hip replacement, though she was young to undergo this type of surgery. (Since artificial hips usually only last for a certain period of time, surgeons prefer to operate on older people and encourage younger people to wait as long as possible.)

From the start, I was suspicious of the diagnosis of hip arthritis. For one thing, the classic symptom of hip arthritis is groin pain—not pain over the outside (lateral) portion of the hip. I examined Margaret and found that she was exquisitely tender over the outside of the hip, which is directly over the trochanteric bursa—a fluid-filled sac that helps to protect joints but can become inflamed and extremely painful for a variety of reasons. Her x-ray showed some mild loss of hip cartilage, which is consistent with a little bit of hip arthritis but generally not enough to cause severe symptoms (though it is well known that patients may experience more severe symptoms than their x-rays would seem to indicate).

After listening to her history, examining her, and reviewing the x-ray of her hip, I concluded that the most likely cause for Margaret's symptoms was *trochanteric bursitis*—a highly treatable condition that usually responds to a number of interventions including physical therapy and corticosteroid injections (sometimes done in a series of two or three). I explained my diagnosis to Margaret and recommended that I inject her hips at that visit; she could then start physical therapy the following week. She agreed and I injected a mixture of anesthetic and corticosteroid into each bursa. By the time she saw the physical therapist her pain had completely resolved. Margaret was elated. She couldn't believe how easy it was to treat her condition. But she was also angry that she had had to live with pain for so long when relief was a simple injection away.

My point in telling Margaret's story is that the *correct* diagnosis is absolutely essential in treating all medical conditions. This example is somewhat unusual in that by the time someone has seen two doctors (including a specialist), she usually has the proper diagnosis. But there are certainly instances in which the appropriate diagnosis is not made, and this can have dramatic consequences for the person suffering from pain. Because establishing the correct diagnosis is the critical first step in treating painful conditions, this chapter is dedicated to reviewing that process.

It's important to note at the outset that many chronic pain conditions are not well understood and may not be able to be precisely diagnosed by even the best specialists. For example, nearly 80 percent of the time doctors are unable to locate the exact cause of low back pain. Although we are learning more each day about what causes a variety of chronic pain conditions, there are still many questions left to answer.

The Black Bag of a Pain Doctor

The diagnostic tools in a pain doctor's black bag are plentiful. They include, among other things, laboratory tests (blood and urine), imaging studies (for example, x-rays and bone scans), and electrophysiologic studies (special nerve and muscle tests). In fact, there are so many different tests that pain doctors spend years learning when to order them, how to interpret them, and then what treatment to recommend. It's not useful in a book like this to go through the litany of tests that a patient might encounter in a chronic pain work-up. More important for the person in pain is to get to the *right* doctor who is skilled at asking the appropriate questions (obtaining a proper medical history is critical in the diagnostic phase of an evaluation), performing a skilled physical examination, ordering the proper tests, and then understanding the results and what should be done next. The first step for the pain patient is to find health-care providers who are experts in the diagnosis of chronic pain conditions.

Primary Care Doctors versus Specialists

Primary care doctors (known as internists, family practitioners, generalists, and pediatricians) are increasingly responsible for diagnosing medical conditions for which they may have had little or no training. Years ago, if someone had a heart condition he was immediately referred to a cardiologist. Now, in the age of managed care, primary care doctors will often treat people who have heart conditions and save the referrals to specialists for the most severe cases. The same is true for many other health problems—including pain.

In the case of chronic pain, it's not unreasonable for primary care doctors to be the first-line resource for patients seeking relief—particularly since the majority of *acute* painful conditions resolve over time without intervention or with very minimal treatment. Although studies show that the majority of patients who seek medical care from a primary care physician report pain as a symptom, most generalists receive very little training in how to diagnose and manage pain. This is a general rule, and there are many exceptions. By definition, however, specialists are doctors who become experts in one particular area of medicine, whereas primary care doctors are generalists who often know a little about a lot of different conditions. Therefore, a referral to a pain specialist is sometimes necessary, and people suffering from chronic pain should know when it's appropriate to obtain a referral and how to ask, or even insist, on seeing a specialist.

In general, if you are having pain, you should first consult your primary care doctor about what's bothering you. If after a month your pain has not *improved* with the treatment your doctor recommends, then it's appropriate to ask to see a specialist. Some primary care doctors will strongly disagree with this statement, and in some instances they would be right. If you have a highly trained primary care doctor who understands a lot about your condition, then it certainly is reasonable to go back to him or her (rather than seeking a consultation with a specialist) and ask for more advice. But if you're suffering and your pain has not improved (most painful conditions will improve, although not necessarily resolve completely, after one month of treatment), then seeing a specialist is entirely appropriate.

Medical doctors who diagnose and treat pain specialize in a number of different fields—physiatry, rheumatology, neurology, and orthopedics. Anesthesiologists are also becoming increasingly interested in pain management, particularly from a procedural point of view (they do a lot of different types of injections and other procedures). There is a great deal of crossover in these specialties, and often any one of several doctors would be a good choice. For example, if you have a rotator cuff tendonitis, a physiatrist, orthopedist, or rheumatologist could effectively diagnose and treat the problem.

Alternative Medicine Practitioners

Seeking a consultation with an alternative medical practitioner who is not a physician is often a thorny issue for chronic pain patients and their families. Many people have very strong views on alternative medicine, and this can result in disagreements among loved ones. In general, my advice is that alternative medicine practitioners should *not* be first-line diagnosticians for the simple fact that they haven't had the training to diagnose complicated medical conditions. Moreover, they are not able to order crucial tests such as MRIs, CT scans, bone scans, and so on. Although some nonphysician practitioners such as chiropractors will order x-rays, they don't have the ability to order or interpret more sophisticated studies. Therefore, I always recommend that people in pain seek a consultation with a physician who is either a medical doctor (M.D.) or an osteopathic doctor (D.O.) specializing in diagnosing chronic pain conditions. In terms of *treatment* (discussed in Chapters 12 and 13), I believe that alternative medicine practitioners have a lot to offer those who suffer from chronic pain.

Individual Doctors versus Pain Clinics

If you are suffering from chronic pain, it really doesn't matter whether you go to an individual doctor or to a pain clinic—the goal is to get to a physician who is knowledgeable and can diagnose your problem. "Pain clinics" can be quite variable in approach, services offered, and expertise available. Some pain clinics will offer excellent diagnostic services, and others won't even have a doctor on staff. Do your research—before making an appointment at a clinic, find out who in your area specializes in diagnosing chronic pain. Clinics typically distinguish themselves on the basis of the type of *treatment* they offer (that is, they generally have a specific focus such as alternative medicine or interventional medicine, focusing on injections). The best pain clinics (discussed in the next two chapters) have comprehensive services and offer many different treatment approaches. Nevertheless, for diagnostic purposes, go to the best doctor you can find who is accessible to you (ideally, someone who is local and is affiliated with your health insurance plan).

Keep in mind that with the billions of consumer and health insurance dollars that are spent on chronic pain each year, this is big business; as such, it attracts many practitioners who call themselves "pain experts." As with anything else, you will find that some of these experts are excellent, some are adequate, and some are wholly unqualified. There are a number of ways you can assess whether a specific practitioner or clinic might be good for you. First, ask your primary care doctor for advice. He is the person you have entrusted to guide you through the medical system, so let him be your guide. Second, contact the American Pain Society or the American Academy of Pain Medicine for information (see the Appendix) and the name of a good pain specialist in your area. Third, consider the fact that doctors and clinics affiliated with accredited medical schools are usually of a fairly high caliber. Be careful when asking friends and family members for advice, especially if they don't have any personal experience with chronic pain or have not done any research.

Sometimes people with chronic pain require hospitalization in order to diagnose the source of their pain. In the acute stage, when pain is new and very severe, there may be a brief hospital stay to help the person manage the pain and to perform a diagnostic work-up quickly. But it's quite rare for someone who has *chronic* pain to be hospitalized in order to run tests and establish the diagnosis. This is simply not cost-effective, and few people want to be hospitalized under these circumstances. Even for treatment, inpatient hospitalizations are rare for people with chronic pain.

Family and the Search for a Diagnosis

Family members often become quite involved in the search for a diagnosis when someone they love is in chronic pain. This can translate into caring and compassionate support for an individual who is suffering, or it can be a terrible burden. Family members can influence a loved one to seek out specialists and multiple consultations and opinions. In some instances, this may lead to a proper diagnosis, effective treatment, and improved quality of life. Unfortunately, in some cases, the family can unwittingly put so much pressure on a loved one that he becomes consumed with the search and has little time for other activities. Even without family pressure, someone can become so obsessed with seeking a diagnosis that he spends an inordinate amount of time doing research on the Internet, participating in online chat rooms, or going from doctor to doctor. It's often hard to know how much to encourage someone in pain to continue the search for a diagnosis. Ideally, the person in pain should pursue appropriate consultations (again, I recommend sticking to physicians who specialize in treating pain for diagnostic evaluations), and family members should be as supportive as possible while at the same time recognizing that the person in pain must ultimately decide what's the best course of action.

12

Traditional Treatment Options

A FIFTY-FOUR-YEAR-OLD man came to see me complaining of hip pain. As I questioned him about his problem it became clear that he only had pain when he crossed his legs in a very awkward position—something he did not routinely do. He further reported that an x-ray of his hip had shown some mild arthritis, and that his primary care doctor had told him that was the cause of his pain. He had insisted on seeing a specialist, and I confirmed what his doctor told him about his diagnosis. He then asked, "What about treatment?" I replied that no treatment was indicated. He appeared confused, but when I elaborated he understood what I meant. Which is this: Painful conditions are treated only when they interfere with someone's ability to do what they want to do, or when they reach a level of discomfort that warrants trying medications (or other treatments) that may pose significant side effects. So in this patient's case, the solution to his pain was not to try medications, injections, or even physical therapy (since he had good range of motion and strength in his hip), but rather to avoid awkwardly crossing his legs. Of course, in the future he might require treatment if his arthritis progresses significantly, but again, treatment should always be based on the current symptoms and limitations that a medical condition poses. At the end of the visit, the man smiled and walked, without a limp or any pain, out of my office.

In contrast to this man who just needed some reassurance, at least once a week I see a patient who has had a serious whiplash (neck) injury as a result of a car accident. The conversation often goes like this:

"So, you were in this car accident two years ago and you've had severe neck pain ever since?"

"Yes."

"And the only treatments you have tried so far are some over-the-counter
medications?"

"Yes."

"Why didn't you try something else?"

"I didn't know that there was anything else I could do, and I was hoping
it would get better on its own."

This conversation highlights a couple of key points. One is that any
pain that lasts longer than one month should be evaluated and treated by
a medical doctor (studies have shown that over 25 percent of chronic
pain sufferers wait at least six months before going to a doctor because
they underestimate the seriousness of the condition and hope it will get
better on its own). Another is that injuries are much easier to treat and
much more responsive to treatment in the early phases. Thus waiting
months or years to treat an injury is not recommended.

Another fairly common scenario is that a patient who was injured several months or even years earlier comes to see me and reports that the
only treatment he has had has been nontraditional in nature (for example, chiropractic, acupuncture, or massage). It's not unusual for these patients to have wiped out their savings on such treatments, since they're
often not covered by medical insurance. Despite knowing how popular
nontraditional treatment options are with the public, I'm always surprised when a patient puts up with months or years' worth of pain and
invests a lot of time and money without trying any of the traditional (and
proven) methods for treating pain. Although nontraditional treatment
can be a very useful adjunct to traditional treatment (and sometimes can
be effective when used alone), it's always worthwhile to consider traditional pain treatment options as a first step (complementary and alternative treatments for pain are discussed in Chapter 13).

Treatment Goals

With many chronic pain conditions a "cure" is not feasible. Treatment focuses on relieving pain as much as possible and improving the patient's
ability to function and quality of life. The goal is to do more and enjoy
more. Treatment also involves educating the patient and the patient's

Non-Pharmacologic Treatment Options for Chronic Pain

Assistive devices (for example, cane)

Biofeedback

Braces

Ergonomic equipment (for example, telephone earset)

Exercise

Footwear/orthotics

Guided imagery

Hypnosis

Massage

Meditation

Modalities such as hot and cold packs

Relaxation therapy

Stress reduction

Transcutaneous electrical nerve stimulation (TENS)

Ultrasound

family about chronic pain and maladaptive pain behaviors, letting them know what therapeutic options are available, and helping them identify ways to modify daily routines to accommodate the condition. Restoring a sense of autonomy, control, and self-esteem is also an integral part of treating chronic pain.

It's important for people in pain and their families to approach treatment with realistic expectations. The physician can help them understand the possible treatment outcomes and what the treatment can and can't do to improve function and reduce pain. Although there are times when a cure is possible—and certainly in the future this will be the case for an increasing number of conditions—for many if not most people with chronic pain, treatment goals are focused on *improving* their level of pain and ability to function.

Traditional Treatment Options

Traditional treatment options in Western medicine generally include therapies that have been scientifically tested and proven to be effective and safe. "Safe" doesn't mean there are no side effects or potential complications; it just means that the benefits of the treatment usually outweigh the associated risks. Some traditional treatments have not undergone rigorous scientific testing but are so widely accepted and used that I include them in this chapter. For the purposes of this chapter I present general categories of traditional treatments without detailing the diagnoses for which they are most appropriate. If you are in pain, discuss these treatment options with your doctor, who can help you decide which therapies are best for your particular condition.

Medications

Medications are often the first-line treatment for chronic pain, and they are usually given in several ways: by mouth (pills), topically (creams or patches), or via injections. The most common oral pain medications include anti-inflammatory drugs, opioids, anti-depressants, muscle relaxants, and anti-convulsants. All these medications have a role in the treatment of chronic pain, but which drugs are most appropriate for a particular person depends on a number of factors, including the underlying medical condition, the type of pain (for example, joint pain, nerve pain), the potential side effects of the medication, and what other drugs the patient is currently taking. How a doctor prescribes medications will

Commonly Used Medications and Their Potential Side Effects

Acetaminophen	liver damage
NSAIDs (nonsteroidal anti-inflammatory drugs)	gastrointestinal bleeding, injury to the kidneys, increased blood pressure
Antidepressants	sedation, dry mouth, constipation, inability to urinate
Muscle relaxants	sedation
Anticonvulsants	dizziness, sedation, constipation, blood or liver injury
Opioids	sedation, nausea, constipation, inability to urinate

also depend on her experience and personal preferences. In addition, the cost of the drug and whether it comes in a less-expensive generic form are considerations for many physicians and patients.

Topical medications can also be useful in treating chronic pain. One of the more common over-the-counter ointments is capsaicin, which is a pepper-based cream. I always recommend that people apply this cream with gloves (so they don't get it on their hands and later touch their eyes) and initially only put it on a very small area, since some people don't like the way it feels. A number of medications are also available as prescription creams and patches. In my practice, I use anesthetic creams and patches as well as special compounds that can be made into a cream by a pharmacist. Opioids can be given topically in patch form as well.

Injections are an excellent way to deliver medications in certain patients. Unfortunately, they are often not used either because the treating physician is not skilled at administering them or because the patient is reluctant to have them. There are many types of injections, but I limit my discussion here to four of the most common and beneficial injections used in treating chronic pain. The first type are *trigger-point injections*. These injections are administered to help relieve muscle pain and typically contain local anesthetic (for example, lidocaine). The injections are done directly into the muscles and away from joints, nerves, and other structures.

The second type of injection contains a mixture of local anesthetic and corticosteroid (for example, "cortisone"). Corticosteriods are produced by our adrenal glands and are among the most powerful anti-inflammatory compounds. They can be given in a variety of medication forms including injections. The benefit of injecting corticosteriods is that the effect will typically be fairly restricted to the injected area. This helps to eliminate some of the problematic side effects that can occur with taking steroids in a pill form (for example, weight gain and bone loss, among others). Injectable corticosteriods are usually quite safe and effective, and they can be used to treat such things as bursitis, tendonitis, nerve injuries, and trigger fingers.

Doctors are discovering the benefits of a third type of injection for pain, botulinum toxin. Initially these injections were used primarily for movement disorders, spasticity, and cosmesis (to lessen wrinkles). Recently, however, there has been good evidence that botulinum toxin works to alleviate pain as well. This makes sense when you consider how it works. Botulinum toxin is produced by the bacteria *Clostridium botulinum* and can be deadly if ingested. The toxin blocks a crucial chemical, acetylcholine, that helps muscles contract. If the availability of this chemical is diminished, then the muscles won't be able to contract with as much force. This is helpful when the muscles are in spasm. Botulinum toxin has been used to treat many painful conditions, including neck and low back pain, buttock pain (piriformis syndrome), headaches (migraines and tension headaches), and facial pain (TMJ). When injected by a doctor skilled in this procedure, it is surprisingly safe and can even be used in people of very advanced age. The effect lasts from weeks to months (usually three to four months), and the injection may or may not need to be repeated, depending on whether the symptoms return.

The fourth type of injections are *spinal injections*, which usually include a mixture of corticosteroid and anesthetic. These injections can be administered in a number of different locations in the spine and are usually identified by the location of the injection (for example, nerve root block, facet block).

There are no hard-and-fast rules for how many of these types of injections a patient can receive, but most physicians will give no more than three injections containing corticosteroid in a twelve-month period in the same location. Trigger-point injections can be given much more frequently. Injections can be extremely helpful in reliving pain and can sometimes even help patients avoid surgery.

Exercise

Exercise is one of the most important methods of treating chronic pain. Many pain situations begin because of muscular imbalance, poor posture, and malalignment of the skeletal structure. For example, people with low back pain often have poor posture, weak abdominal muscles, and tight hamstring muscles. In physical therapy, a patient with this condition will typically be given a "lumbar stabilization" exercise program that will address all these problems. Even if someone develops pain after an injury, the recovery may be prolonged as a result of pre-existing muscular imbalances. Moreover, people with chronic pain tend to become increasingly sedentary, which leads to physical deconditioning and eventu-

Common Types of Pain Treatment Injections

Trigger-point injections	Administered in specific areas of the muscle that are pain generators (fibromyalgia, myofascial pain syndromes, etc.).
Tendon injections	Medication is injected around, but not into, the tendon (tendonitis, lateral epicondylitis, etc.).
Nerve blocks	Medication is injected near the nerve but not into the nerve (reflex sympathetic dystrophy, carpal tunnel syndrome, spinal nerve compression syndromes, etc.).
Epidural injections	Medication is delivered to the epidural space in the spine (spinal stenosis, lumbar, or cervical radiculopathy from a herniated disk).
Facet blocks	Injections are performed in the facet joints in the spine for relief of pain usually due to arthritis of the facet joint itself (cervical facet arthropathy, lumbar facet joint pain).
Botulinum toxin injections	Botulinum toxin is injected directly into the muscles to decrease muscle spasm or spasticity (stroke, multiple sclerosis, migraine headaches, etc.).
Joint injections	Medication is injected into the joint space (knee arthritis, sacroiliac joint pain, etc.).
Bursitis injections	If the bursa is inflamed, the first part of the procedure may involve draining the fluid and the second part injecting medication to reduce inflammation (shoulder bursitis, hip bursitis, etc.).

ally even more pain. Exercise also has enormous psychological benefits that can enhance someone's ability to function.

When treating chronic pain, doctors often send patients to physical and/or occupational therapy to learn specific exercises. Because many conditions can worsen with the wrong type of exercise, I typically refer patients to expert therapists who can address their particular problem.

There are different types of exercises (flexibility, strengthening, and cardiovascular or aerobic), and a good therapist can help create a program that incorporates specific exercises from each category to promote reconditioning and healing. As with all professions, therapists vary in their skill levels and interests, so be sure to find someone who is accustomed to dealing with chronic pain and is skilled at treating people with your particular condition. I usually encourage patients who are very sedentary to begin exercising on their own at the same time as they begin physical therapy—even if it just means a five-minute walk. As a cautionary note, you should always check with your doctor before beginning any exercise program—this is particularly important for people with a history of heart disease.

Modalities

Modalities are treatments that are applied to a painful area on the body, such as hot or cold packs—which can both be used at home. It's important to note that both heat and cold can cause serious tissue damage if applied for too long or at very extreme temperatures. Neither hot nor cold packs should be directly applied to the skin. Cold packs should not be left on for more than twenty minutes at a time, with at least an hour break in between treatments. In addition, cold packs should not be applied to the extremities in people who have problems with circulation (for example, peripheral vascular disease).

Ice massage can also be an effective method of relieving pain. You can do this yourself by freezing a paper cup filled with water and cutting the cup to expose the ice. Then apply the ice to the affected area in a circular motion. Another home-based remedy is transcutaneous electrical nerve stimulation (TENS), which is a unit with electrodes that stick to the skin. This unit is first used in physical therapy to assess whether it's helpful in relieving the pain, and if so it's then given to someone to use at home. TENS units are small and compact (similar to a cell phone) and can be easily hidden under clothes. They are typically worn intermittently during the day. Interferential units are similar to TENS but are usually used for acute pain. Occasionally they are used for chronic pain but tend to work better for acute pain issues such as the reduction of edema.

Other modalities are more sophisticated and require special training on the part of therapists. These can include electrical stimulation, ultrasound (a deep heating method), and iontophoresis and phonophoresis (both of which can be used to help topically applied corticosteroids penetrate the skin without breaking it as an injection does). In people with dark skin, corticosteroids (whether applied on the surface of the skin or beneath the surface), can cause lightening of the skin in the region where they're used. Other precautions should be taken with different modalities (for example, ultrasound should not be used directly over cemented joint replacements), and the prescribing physician and therapist should be aware of these.

Physical and occupational therapists often perform what is generally termed "manual therapy." This therapy includes joint-mobilization techniques to aid with pain reduction through normalizing the alignment of bones and the surrounding soft tissues. Myofascial release techniques further help to normalize soft tissue and can lead to pain relief. These include craniosacral therapy, deep-tissue massage, and muscle triggerpoint massage.

Special Equipment

There are many pieces of equipment that can help with pain relief depending on the particular condition. For example, a telephone headset or earset is ideal for someone with neck pain. If you have hand pain and need to use the computer, voice-activated software can be a lifesaver. If you have back pain or foot pain, custom shoe orthotics and/or extra-depth and -width orthopedic shoes can provide relief. If you have hip or knee pain, a cane can help unload the affected joint and thereby lessen the pain. In fact, there are so many types of equipment that it's impossible to discuss them all here. The important thing is to get the right equipment to treat your particular condition.

Frank, a long-standing patient of mine, discovered the importance of the right equipment when he came to see me with severe ankle arthritis that made every step excruciating. Frank told me that he had been to see an orthopedic surgeon who had recommended an ankle fusion to relieve the pain. Frank had decided against the surgery, because he had significant heart disease and was worried he wouldn't make it through the operation. I told Frank that there was a good chance he could be fit with a special brace (called an ankle foot orthosis, or AFO) that would completely relieve his pain. Frank was doubtful that this would help, but when he came to our brace clinic and tried out the brace, he couldn't believe that all his pain disappeared. I just saw Frank again recently, and he has been walking pain-free for more than a year with his new brace.

This example illustrates the importance of the right equipment in successfully treating chronic pain. It also shows that getting a second opinion from a doctor who specializes in treating chronic pain in a different medical specialty can provide additional treatment options.

Lifestyle Changes

Linda is a pediatrician who works in an office with a tile floor. She and many of her colleagues have chronic foot pain (plantar fasciitis) caused and exacerbated by standing all day on this unforgiving surface. There are a number of ways to treat this condition, but one of the most effective is to eliminate or at least modify whatever is causing the pain (in this case, standing on the tile floor). Two relatively easy lifestyle modifications for Linda would be to obtain "stress mats" (cushioned surfaces that are widely available in stores that sell kitchen mats) to stand on at work, and to sit down whenever possible.

Sometimes people have to go to extraordinary lengths to alter their lifestyle in order to decrease pain. For example, one of my patients who complained of neck and shoulder pain had to quit her job and seek alternative employment when she realized that no amount of physical therapy, medication, or other treatments would alleviate her pain so long as she continued carrying heavy suitcases and a laptop computer and sitting for long hours on transatlantic flights.

When I talk to patients about lifestyle modifications, the first thing I ask is, "What are you doing that worsens the pain?" I'm often surprised at how many people have not taken the time to think about how their daily activities relate to their pain. This can be an extremely useful exercise. If you have pain, start by assessing what you are physically doing that makes it worse. Then look for solutions to modify those activities.

Psychological Intervention

I recently sent one of my patients for a consultation with a colleague who specializes in treating chronic pain. The patient was complaining of severe hand pain but had no objective findings (his physical examination, x-rays, and lab tests were all completely normal). My colleague concurred with the results of my work-up—that there was no identifiable reason for this man's pain. Yet we both believed that this patient was suffering. In order to help him, my colleague suggested a psychiatric consultation to evaluate and treat the patient's anxiety. In explaining the reason for the referral to my patient, I told him that we did not believe the pain was "all in his head" but that his overall anxiety was lessening his ability to cope with the pain. Indeed, once his anxiety was under control, despite continued hand pain, he felt much better.

In chronic pain treatment programs, a clinical social worker, psychologist, or psychiatrist will often participate in helping both the patient and the family deal with the emotional aspects of the problem. Psychiatrists usually focus on prescribing medications that will help improve depression and anxiety. Clinical social workers and psychologists can provide counseling and may use techniques such as guided imagery, hypnosis, and therapeutic touch to decrease stress and improve the patient's ability to deal with pain. The treatment usually also involves learning healthy ways of communicating with loved ones and avoiding chronic pain behaviors. Mental health professionals also address issues related to low self-esteem. The family may be involved in some of the sessions to learn ways to help their loved one with maladaptive pain behaviors and other issues surrounding chronic pain.

Surgery

Surgery is an excellent method of treatment for some chronic pain problems; however, because of the potential for serious side effects, patients should first explore other options. Many patients turn to surgeons before consulting other doctors, but it's important to recognize that surgeons rely heavily on operations as a method of treating pain (in medical school we would say the surgeon's motto is "a chance to cut is a chance to cure"). This overstates the case, of course; many surgeons are very conservative and use operations only as a "last resort." Moreover, surgery is absolutely appropriate in certain cases. But often there are nonsurgical options that patients should consider. For example, I see hundreds of patients each year with "herniated discs" in their backs. Many people mistakenly believe that surgery is the only option for this problem. In fact, surgery is indicated for disc problems only if the disc: (1) causes severe intractable pain that is not responsive to conservative (nonsurgical) treatment; (2) is associated with weakness due to pressure on a nerve; or (3) causes bowel or bladder problems.

If you're considering surgery for a chronic pain problem, think about consulting a doctor who specializes in chronic pain but does not perform surgery. There may be other, less risky treatment options available to you.

Pain Clinics

In a 1999 survey sponsored by the American Pain Society, only 22 percent of participants reported that they had been referred to a specialized treatment program for their pain.[1] Deciding whether to go to a pain clinic and which one to attend can be a difficult and confusing process. If you're considering seeking treatment at a pain clinic (also known as a pain center or program), find out first which services the facility offers (see the Appendix). Many pain clinics have a specific focus (complementary and alternative medicine, medical management with medications only, or injection therapy). Focused pain clinics can be helpful if the type of pain you have usually responds to the treatment offered. Often, however, services at very focused clinics will not provide enough depth to help individuals who are suffering from chronic pain. Therefore, you might want to consider going to a pain clinic that offers a variety of treatment options with a multidisciplinary staff. These types of pain clinics can be hard to find but are well worth the effort. To research where you might find one, contact the American Pain Association and other organizations listed in the Appendix. You can also ask your doctor or other healthcare professionals for advice. Your local hospital will provide information on the clinics it offers. In addition, check with family members and friends who may have personal experience with a particular pain clinic. The Internet is a wonderful resource as well, but be sure you double-check any information to be sure it's legitimate.

Special Considerations for Children

One of my colleagues received a call from the school nurse at her son's kindergarten. The nurse reported that her child was too tired to stay awake in class. On her way to pick him up, my colleague called her husband and discovered that they had both been giving him his allergy medication (thus doubling his dose). At the advice of their pediatrician, they stopped the medication altogether for a few days and then resumed his usual dose without any undue side effects.

This episode illustrates a couple of considerations that are unique to children. First, young children typically don't know how much medication they are supposed to take and therefore will not be able to monitor their own intake. This can lead to confusion for parents if they don't have a set system in place. Even with a system, it's often hard to decide whether to give a child medication for pain, since they can't always articulate their symptoms. Subtle behavioral changes may be the only evidence of worsening pain. Even with older children and teens who are able to take their own medications, parents need to monitor the process to ensure that the correct amount is taken. Second, children don't always mention medication side effects, and it's not unusual for parents to attribute observed side effects to other things. For instance, my colleague immediately assumed that her son was staying up too late at night or was coming down with an illness—it was only after she had talked to her husband that she even considered medication side effects as the culprit in her child's fatigue. Side effects can present as medical emergencies when they are not caught early; for instance, constipation from opioids can lead to bowel obstruction. Parents should also be aware that medication side effects may be different in children than in adults. For example, infants are not able to eliminate drugs in the same way that adults can because of the immaturity of their kidneys, and medications that are usually sedating can paradoxically cause a child to become hyperactive in some cases. Third, some medications that adults use routinely should not be given to children. An example of such a medication is aspirin, which on rare occasions can be quite harmful to children.

Whenever a child enters the medical system, he or she loses control, and it's important for parents and caregivers to understand this—particularly if a child is facing surgery or a hospitalization. The more you explain the treatment and the treatment *process* to your child, the better. There are several excellent children's books on hospitalization and surgery that can help. When treating children for chronic pain, it's important to address their psychological health and social adjustment as well. There are a number of ways to do this, including through "play therapy," which provides a safe environment for children to communicate anxiety, fear, and sadness. Other special considerations in the pediatric population include the fact that children who use special equipment will outgrow it (sometimes fairly quickly), which can be costly (shoe orthotics and braces, for example, need to be changed at least once a year). Children can benefit from stress-reduction and relaxation techniques, but they may not be able to participate at a young age. Moreover, older children are not always compliant when it comes to exercise and lifestyle adjustments.

Special Considerations for Older Individuals

Physicians must consider a number of medication-related issues when treating pain in older people. First, older individuals often have more advanced disease than younger patients (osteoarthritis, for example, is usually more severe in an eighty-year-old than in someone who is forty) and thus more pain. Additionally, pain in the advanced stage of an illness may be more refractory to treatment. Second, there are many more opportunities for elders to have pain owing to specific illnesses or normal aging of the body. Young people usually have one chronic pain problem, but older individuals may have several. Third, medications may be less effective in the elderly because of changes in blood flow to organs and other body changes that occur with aging. Or the potential side effects might be more pronounced. Moreover, prescription options are sometimes limited because a patient is already on multiple different medications. In fact, the average seventy-year-old takes seven different medications, thus increasing the risk of serious drug interactions. Doctors need to know not only the prescription medications someone is using but also all the over-the-counter remedies she is taking.

A fourth factor to consider in medication use among seniors is the cost. The cost of medications for those on a fixed income can be prohibitively expensive, and so they may not take their medications as prescribed. If this is the case, then obviously the treatment may not be very effective. Fifth, anxiety and depression are common but often overlooked in older patients. Their ability to focus mentally may be impaired as a result of emotional issues or secondary to dementia. It can be difficult to treat people who can't concentrate well because they are unable to participate fully in the treatment. Medication to alleviate anxiety and depression can be very helpful in the treatment of chronic pain in elders.

Nonmedication issues also factor into treatment for people of advanced age. For example, studies reveal that older people tend to be less active, and with decreased activity comes more pain. Even moderate physical exercise can play a preventative and possibly a restorative role when it comes to certain types of pain, including osteoarthritis. The skeletal structure of older individuals is also more fragile than that of younger patients (often as a result of osteoporosis), so treatment prescriptions such as physical therapy should take this into account. Finally, elderly individuals may have fewer treatment options owing to their age and physical health (for example, severe heart disease may render surgery too high a risk).

Family members can help an older loved one in a variety of ways. Of course, just being a sympathetic listener and acknowledging that aging can be difficult is important. More concrete ways of providing assistance might include typing up your loved one's medical history so he has it readily available to take to doctors' appointments. In the same vein, you could type up a list of medications, including the name of the drug, the dose, and how often it is taken. If your loved one is searching for a pain doctor or pain clinic, you can help by consulting the Appendix in this book, making calls to surrounding hospitals, or searching the Internet. You might offer to drive a loved one to medical or therapy appointments. The occupational therapists at my center frequently visit older people's homes to assist them in making their environment safer. Often their homes are hazardous owing to all the clutter that has accumulated as they've become more frail and unable to do a lot of lifting or heavy cleaning. Thus helping to clean up will make a loved one's home not only more pleasant but also safer. These are just a few suggestions, of course —there are numerous ways you can help an older loved one cope with chronic pain.

13

Complementary and Alternative Medicine

COMPLEMENTARY and alternative medicine (CAM) includes a wide variety of treatments that are by definition not part of conventional medicine. Common CAM therapies used in the treatment of chronic pain include chiropractic manipulation, acupuncture, massage, and homeopathy. The National Center for Complementary and Alternative Medicine (NCCAM), part of the National Institutes of Health (NIH), defines CAM as "a group of diverse medical and healthcare systems, practices and products that are not presently considered to be part of conventional medicine."

Although complementary and alternative treatments are grouped together under the rubric CAM, there is actually a clear distinction between them: complementary refers to those treatments that are used together with conventional medical therapies, whereas alternative medicine refers to treatments used in place of conventional treatments. CAM therapies are sometimes referred to as "holistic" or "integrative." Holistic treatment approaches involve caring for the whole person (body, mind, emotions, and spirit), and integrative therapies are those treatments that fall into the category of holistic care. For the purposes of this discussion, I'll use the general term CAM and note any important distinctions among therapies.

NCCAM divides treatments into five basic categories or domains. These include: (1) alternative medical systems, including homeopathic and naturopathic medicine; (2) mind-body interventions that include meditation and prayer; (3) biologically based therapies such as herbs and other dietary supplements that are found in nature; (4) manipulative and body-based methods, including massage therapy and osteopathic and

Some CAM Therapies

Acupuncture
Applied kinesiology
Aromatherapy
Ayurvedic medicine
Biofeedback
Biological dentistry
Bodywork
Chelation therapy
Chiropractic treatment
Craniosacral therapy
Energy medicine
Environmental medicine
Guided imagery
Herbal medicine
Homeopathy
Hydrotherapy
Light therapy
Magnetic field therapy
Massage
Mind-body medicine
Natural hormone replacement therapy
Naturopathic medicine
Neural therapy
Nutritional medicine
Orthomolecular medicine
Osteopathic medicine
Oxygen therapies
Prolotherapy
Qigong and Tai chi
Sound therapy
Traditional Chinese medicine
Yoga

chiropractic manipulation; and (5) energy therapies such as therapeutic touch and magnets.

CAM treatments, and people's interest in them, are growing by leaps and bounds. It's estimated that at least two-thirds of Americans have tried CAM, and each year more than twenty-five billion dollars is spent on these therapies in the United States. Some studies have shown that more than 50 percent of mainstream doctors have tried CAM themselves, and a similar number have reported recommending CAM therapies to their patients. Physicians tend to favor chiropractic, acupuncture, biofeedback, massage, relaxation, and nutritional supplements. In a study conducted in 2002, 84 percent of the doctors surveyed reported thinking that they needed to learn more about CAM to adequately address patient concerns. Most medical doctors have not had formal training in CAM, though this situation is beginning to change as Western medical schools adopt CAM as part of their curricula.

There are clear trends in CAM use. For instance, women use CAM more frequently than men, and CAM therapies are more common in younger and middle-aged individuals than in children and the elderly. Approximately 20–30 percent of general pediatric patients have tried at least one CAM therapy, and in teens that number may be as high as 50–75 percent. In one study, mothers who took their children to CAM providers were more likely to be over thirty-one years of age, religious, born outside of the United States, or CAM users themselves. In this same study, the most common treatments tried were herbs, prayer healing, and high-dose vitamins and other nutritional supplements. Older individuals also use CAM, though somewhat less frequently (in one study of older Americans 41 percent of respondents reported using CAM, with herbs, chiropractic, massage, and acupuncture being the most frequently cited therapies). Interestingly, those who use CAM therapies tend to have moderate to high levels of income and education. Studies also reveal, however, that the majority of patients who use CAM do not report this to their doctors.

CAM is an important option for people with chronic pain who have not responded to conventional medicine. But before deciding if unconventional treatments are right for you, you should understand this diverse and often misused and misunderstood group of treatment options.

The CAM Controversy

In the past, CAM treatments had virtually no proven effects. This is not to say that they didn't work, but simply that they hadn't been studied in the way that we study conventional medical treatments. Because conventional medicine is "evidence-based," meaning that medical doctors usually don't prescribe treatments for patients unless they are proven to be beneficial, this lack of research has led to enormous controversy. Some alternative healthcare providers have taken advantage of people who are ill and desperate by giving them CAM treatments that are costly, not covered by medical insurance, unhelpful, and sometimes even harmful. Moreover, there are tremendous marketing forces at work for CAM treatments. For example, doctors have recognized that eating yogurt can help with diarrhea. This finding has led health food stores to stock many products with similar ingredients (primarily lactobacillus bacteria) that claim to "support healthy intestinal function." The effectiveness and safe dosing for nearly all of these products are not known.

As a teenager I remember my mother telling me that when she was young people believed tobacco was harmless. I was shocked and kept asking her how they could possibly have believed that such a toxic substance could be safe. The answer, of course, was that people had used tobacco for centuries for medicinal, recreational, and religious purposes without recognizing the *cumulative* hazards associated with chronic use. Thus to say that it's safe to use products that have not been scientifically studied is not accurate. It may be safe to use them or it may not.

On the other hand, there are certainly instances where CAM therapies provide pain relief. Although up to 80 percent of people who have tried CAM report at least some relief, it's impossible to determine whether the therapies really work without controlled scientific studies that look beyond the placebo effect. The medical community as a whole has come to recognize that some (but certainly not all) of these nontraditional therapies may significantly improve people's health. The NCCAM was created to determine which of these treatments are effective by using controlled scientific studies to determine their benefits (and potential harmful side effects). Many other organizations and researchers share this mission. Significantly, as CAM treatments are proven to be safe and effective they are sometimes adopted into conventional healthcare.

CAM and Chronic Pain

As an allopathic physician (one trained in the Western tradition) who believes that some CAM treatments can be very helpful, I always tell my patients in pain that it's imperative to initially seek a diagnosis from a conventional doctor who is an expert in pain medicine. Only conventionally trained doctors have the skills and ability to use the latest technology to evaluate a medical problem. This does not mean that CAM practitioners are not skilled diagnosticians—some of them may be quite expert. But even if your massage therapist or chiropractor is excellent, he or she is not able to order blood tests or imaging studies such as MRIs that may identify the cause of your symptoms. I always tell my patients that we need a diagnosis before prescribing appropriate treatment—regardless of whether the treatment involves conventional medicine and/or CAM.

Of course, there are many times in the chronic pain field when a specific diagnosis is not clear. Whenever someone has pain without a clear diagnosis, I always want to know what work-up has been done and if it was sufficient. If it was not sufficient, then further tests are indicated. If an exhaustive investigation has been done and the most serious conditions have been ruled out but there still is not a clear diagnosis, then I recommend that treatment be initiated to give the patient some relief.

Once someone is ready to begin the treatment phase, I always suggest that the conventional doctor be kept "in the loop." This will ensure that the patient understands the options, benefits, and risks of conventional treatment. For example, I have had a number of patients come to me with very severe carpal tunnel syndrome (in this condition, the median nerve at the wrist is compressed by the wrist structures, which can lead to permanent loss of hand function). In most instances, they knew they had carpal tunnel syndrome but decided to try alternative medicine therapies such as acupuncture, massage, and herbs rather than conventional therapies such as anti-inflammatory medications, wrist splints, injections, and surgery. Unfortunately, by the time they saw me, they had suffered permanent hand paralysis and numbness to the point where they were seriously impaired. Although they all ultimately underwent surgical release of the nerve, the operation was performed simply to prevent further injury—they still were left with serious deficits.

The take-home message here is that only a medical doctor has the knowledge and ability definitively to diagnose carpal tunnel syndrome by doing electrodiagnostic testing (which is very sensitive and positively identifies carpal tunnel syndrome without a doubt in most cases) and then to inform a patient what the current scientific literature says about how to treat this condition. In fact, research supports surgery in most cases of severe carpal tunnel syndrome because it's the only way to relieve the pressure from the nerve and prevent further injury (mild and moderate carpal tunnel syndrome can often be treated without surgery). The patients I have seen with severe carpal tunnel syndrome who first tried alternative therapies all have serious regrets about the fact that they delayed getting information about the seriousness of this condition and the treatment options that have been proven to work. So my advice is this: Though it's fine to explore and even try CAM therapies, don't neglect to get information about your condition and what treatments have been proven to work, or at least have been proven to have significant benefit.

CAM therapies such as acupuncture, massage, biofeedback, and chiropractic and osteopathic manipulation have been shown to have therapeutic benefit in selected chronic pain patients. Moreover, most doctors who specialize in treating chronic pain regularly prescribe at least some CAM treatments. In fact, the treatments listed above, though still considered CAM, are becoming so integrated into the treatment of chronic pain patients at pain centers that they really occupy a gray area where CAM and conventional medicine intersect. On the other hand, there are many CAM therapies that are not embraced by the medical community and may even be harmful in some instances.

Special Considerations for Children

CAM is becoming increasingly popular in children and teens; however, it's important to note a few special considerations in these populations. Perhaps the most concerning issue has to do with medications and nutritional supplements that are readily available in health food stores, drug stores, and supermarkets, or for sale over the Internet. The problem is that for the vast majority of these supplements, there are no available data to show that they work in children or are safe for children to use.

Children, with their immature skeletal systems and other organs, may be more susceptible to serious side effects (for example, growth retardation) than teens and adults. The fact that the dosing is very inconsistent further complicates matters, as do herb-drug interactions that can occur in children who are also taking prescription medications. Despite these problems, there is an enormous effort being made to market pediatric herbal products and other supplements.

Preliminary studies have shown that lifestyle therapies such as mind-body medicine, which can involve hypnosis, can prevent migraines and reduce pain and nausea from chemotherapy in children. Massage has been used for pain and depression (as well as to help newborns gain weight and to treat asthma, attention deficit hyperactivity disorder, and so on). Massage is enjoyable and safe for most children. Acupuncture may provide the same proven therapeutic benefit for children as it does for adults, but the trauma of the needles may limit this as a treatment option.

Special Considerations for Older Individuals

Nutritional supplements are also a major concern for older pain sufferers. For example, St. John's Wort, an herb used for pain and depression, is known to lower the blood levels of the prescription medication digoxin, which is commonly used by older individuals who have heart problems. Thus someone using St. John's Wort and digoxin may suffer from a life-threatening cardiac problem because the digoxin is not at the level it needs to be. St. John's Wort can also interfere with other medications, as can many other herbs and supplements. Because older people often take many more medications than younger people, the chance for interactions and side effects is much greater. Aging also affects how drugs and other supplements are eliminated from the body; thus a drug that's tolerated just fine by a forty-year-old may cause serious toxicity in an eighty-year-old.

Aggressive massage therapy and spinal manipulation should not be performed on anyone who is frail and susceptible to bony fractures from osteoporosis. Exercises done without consulting a doctor can exacerbate an underlying heart or lung condition—which can be disastrous in older individuals. Prayer, meditation, and hypnosis might not be options in someone who is suffering from pain and dementia. Acupuncture has been shown to be a safe and useful adjunct to mainstream therapies.

CAM and the Family

At a dinner gathering of college friends, the attendees were remembering with fondness a classmate who had recently died of breast cancer. A former roommate who had lived with her for many years lamented that she had not tried alternative therapies when she learned of her terminal diagnosis. "If only she had at least *tried* something else," she said. Family members and friends often have extreme views on CAM. Some strongly advocate for it even when it doesn't make any sense (as is the case, nearly always, when looking for a "cure" in terminal cancer), whereas others don't believe that any CAM treatments are appropriate under any circumstances. I counsel patients and families to take a moderate approach, especially in chronic pain, which can significantly improve with some CAM therapies, and to use the criteria listed in the next section as a means of determining whether to try a specific CAM therapy.

Choosing CAM Treatments and Practitioners

When I first began practicing medicine, one of the older doctors in my practice encouraged me to do some "peer review" to further my education. This involved reviewing the charts of other doctors and generating a report that either concurred with their recommended treatment or provided reasons the treatment was not appropriate. In mainstream medicine this is a common practice and is sometimes referred to as "utilization review." The goal is to make sure that the prescribed treatment is reasonable on the basis of scientific studies and the "standard of care" in a given geographic region. What I found was that most mainstream doctors were prescribing treatment very appropriately. One doctor who worked at a pain clinic, though, sent every patient he saw for chiropractic treatment. In one case, a five-year-old boy came in with a stiff neck and sore throat about one week after being involved in a car accident. His mother told the doctor that he had been sick, and this was noted in the records. The doctor performed a perfunctory and incomplete examination of the boy that did not include taking his temperature and checking his neck movement, which are critical steps in assessing whether a child with a stiff neck might have meningitis—a potentially deadly disease. As with every other case I reviewed on this doctor, the boy was sent to a chiropractor in the same facility. On the initial evaluation a few days later, the chiropractor noted that the child was "asymptomatic," but he still treated him with spinal manipulation for several weeks. Needless to say, I concluded that the diagnostic work-up was flawed and that the treatment was not appropriate. A few weeks after I submitted my report, I began receiving threatening phone calls from an administrator at the pain clinic. I contacted a federal prosecutor at the United States Attorney's Office in Boston and learned that this entire group was under investigation and that criminal action was imminent.

My purpose in relaying this story is to tell readers to trust their instincts. Regardless of who is making the recommendations, do they make sense? Do you have confidence in how the specialist evaluated you and the treatment that he or she recommended? If you're considering CAM therapies (this is also true for mainstream medicine), then it's important for you to understand as much as you can about the treatment. You'll want to know the following:

1. Is this treatment safe for my medical condition and for me as an individual?
2. Is there a good chance that this treatment will be effective in my case?
3. What will the total cost of the treatment be?
4. Is the practitioner I plan to use an expert in this field?
5. What does my doctor think about my trying this treatment?

You can answer most of these questions by talking to your doctor and doing a little research on your own. One of the most reliable places to look for information on CAM is the NCCAM, which is sponsored by the United States government. Contact information for NCCAM is listed in the Appendix.

Whether or not you decide to try a CAM treatment, remember—*never substitute an unproven treatment for a proven one.*

Afterword

MEDICINE is a constantly changing and evolving field, but one fact remains indisputable—no one chooses to become sick. Rather, illness chooses us, often despite our best efforts to eat properly, exercise regularly, and live a "healthy" life. If you've read this book, chances are you or someone you love suffers chronic pain. Your choice, then, is not whether chronic pain exists in your life, but rather *how you are going to react to it*. Will pain control you and your family, or will you find a way to live a meaningful life *despite* the pain? Virginia Woolf wrote, "Considering how common illness is, how tremendous the spiritual change that it brings, how astonishing, when the lights of health go down, the undiscovered countries that are then disclosed."[1] Chronic pain offers you a unique perspective—a special lens from which to view the landscape of your life.

Although pain may have left its indelible mark on you, there are good reasons to be hopeful about the future. Doctors and scientists are working hard to find better treatments and even cures for chronic pain conditions. It's heartening to witness how some of these treatments become available seemingly overnight. For example, when I began writing this book, botulinum toxin was a drug that doctors used to treat wrinkles and spasticity. As I write this Afterword, numerous studies have demonstrated that botulinum toxin is very effective for a variety of pain conditions. One of my patients, a lovely fifty-five-year-old woman with chronic neck pain, had tried virtually every type of treatment available over the twenty years she has been suffering with pain. A few months ago I suggested botulinum toxin, and it worked beautifully. She is pain-free for the first time in more than two decades. My patient thinks it's a miracle, but really it's just the culmination of years of research by many dedicated scientists working to alleviate certain types of pain.

I have witnessed many wonderful cures in medicine—including in people who have lived with chronic pain for years. Because of this, I maintain tremendous hope for the future. This is not to say that we don't have some very effective therapies right now—indeed we do. If you or a loved one is in pain, continue to explore reasonable treatment options. At the same time, I encourage you to practice "mindfulness," that is, try to make the most of your life right now—despite whatever hardships you are enduring. Of course, when you're suffering this can be difficult to do. But you and your loved ones will benefit tremendously if you refuse to let pain control your life and inform your decisions. In her autobiography Margiad Evans wrote, "Our health is a voyage: and every illness is an adventure story."[2] Let the adventure begin.

Resources

GENERAL RESOURCES

Addiction Resource Guide
P.O. Box 8612
Tarrytown, NY 10591
(914) 725-5151
www.addictionresourceguide.com

American Chronic Pain Association
P.O. Box 850
Rocklin, CA 95677
(916) 632-0922
www.theacpa.org
e-mail: acpa@pacbell.net

American Pain Society
4700 West Lake Avenue
Glenview, IL 60025
(847) 375-4715
www.ampainsoc.org
e-mail: info@ampainsoc.org

American Psychiatric Association
1000 Wilson Boulevard
Suite 1825
Arlington, VA 22209-3901
1-888-35-PSYCH
www.psych.org

American Psychological Association
750 First Street, N.E.
Washington, D.C. 20002-4242
1-800-374-2721
www.apa.org

American Society of Addiction Medicine (ASAM)
4601 North Park Avenue
Arcate Suite 101
Chevy Chase, MD 20815
(301) 656-3920
www.asam.org

Council of State Administrators of Vocational Rehabilitation (CSAVR)
4733 Bethesda Avenue
Suite 330
Bethesda, MD 20814
(301) 654-8414
www.rehabnetwork.org

Narcotics Anonymous (NA)
P.O. Box 9999
Van Nuys, CA 91409
(818) 773-9999
www.na.org

National Association of Social Workers
750 First Street, N.E.
Suite 700
Washington, D.C. 20002-4241
(202) 408-8600
www.socialworkers.org

National Center for Complementary and Alternative Medicine (NCCAM)
P.O. Box 7923
Gaithersburg, MD 20898
1-888-644-6226
www.nccam.nih.gov

National Family Caregivers Association
10605 Concord Street, Suite 501
Kensington, MD 20895
1-800-896-3650
www.nfcacares.org
e-mail: info@nfcacares.org

National Institute on Drug Abuse (NIDA)
National Institutes of Health
9000 Rockville Pike
Bethesda, MD 20892
www.drugabuse.gov/NIDAHome

The National Pain Foundation
P.O. Box 102605
Denver, CO 80250
www.painconnection.com
e-mail: aardrup@painconnection.org

Prescription Anonymous, Inc.
P.O. Box 10534
Gaithersburg, MD 10534
www.prescriptionanonymous.org

Sex Information and Education Council of the United States
130 West 42nd Street
Suite 350
New York, NY 10036-7802
(212) 819-9770
www.siecus.org

The Well Spouse Foundation
P.O. Box 30093
Elkins Park, NJ 07728
1-800-838-0879
www.wellspouse.org
e-mail: info@wellspouse.org

RESOURCES FOR FINDING CHRONIC PAIN TREATMENT

American Academy of Pain Medicine
4700 West Lake Avenue
Glenview, IL 60025
(847) 375-4777
www.painmed.org

American Academy of Physical Medicine and Rehabilitation (AAPM&R)
One IBM Plaza
Suite 2500
Chicago, IL 60611-3604
(312) 464-9700
www.aapmr.org

American Chronic Pain Association
PO Box 850
Rocklin, CA 95677
(916) 632-0922
www.theacpa.org

Commission on Accreditation of Rehabilitation Facilities (CARF)
4891 East Grant Road
Tucson, AZ 85712
(520) 325-1044
www.carf.org

Joint Commission on Accreditation of Healthcare Organizations (JCAHO)
One Renaissance Blvd.
Oakbrook Terrace, IL 60181
(630) 792-5000
www.jcaho.org

Suggested Reading

THE HISTORY OF PAIN

Good, Mary-Jo Delvecchio, et al. *Pain as Human Experience: An Anthropological Perspective*. Berkeley, Calif.: University of California Press, 1994.

Kleinman, Arthur. *The Illness Narratives: Suffering, Healing and the Human Condition*, New York: Basic Books, 1988.

Morris, David B. *The Culture of Pain*. Berkeley, Calif.: University of California Press, 1991.

Rey, Roselyne. *The History of Pain*, trans. Louise Elliot Wallace, J. A. Cadden, and S. W. Cadden. Cambridge, Mass.: Harvard University Press, 1995.

Vertosick, Frank T., Jr. *Why We Hurt: The Natural History of Pain*. Orlando, Fla.: Harcourt, Inc., 2000.

Wall, Patrick. *Pain: The Science of Suffering*. New York: Columbia University Press, 2000.

PAIN AND THE FAMILY

Cowan, Penney. *Family Manual: A Manual for Families of Persons with Pain*, ed. Nicole Kelly, Christine Pasero, Edward Covington, and Charles Lidz. Rocklin, Calif.: American Chronic Pain Association, Inc., 1998.

Goldenberg, Don L. *Chronic Illness and Uncertainty: A Personal Guide to Poorly Understood Syndromes*. Newton Upper Falls, Mass.: Dorset Press, 1996.

McDaniel, Susan H., Jeri Hepworth, and William J. Doherty. *Medical Family Therapy: A Biopsychological Approach to Families with Health Problems*, New York: Basic Books, 1992.

McLeod, Beth Witrogen. *Caregiving: The Spiritual Journey of Love, Loss, and Renewal*. New York: Wiley and Sons, 1999.

Miller, James E. *When You're the Caregiver: Twelve Things to Do if Someone You Care for Is Ill or Incapacitated*. Fort Wayne, Ind.: Willowgreen Publishing, 1995.

Miller, Judith Fitzgerald. *Coping with Chronic Illness: Overcoming Powerlessness*, 3rd ed. Philadelphia, Penn.: F. A. Davis Company, 2000.

Welsh, Linda, and Marian Betancourt. *Chronic Illness and the Family: A Guide for Living*. Holbrook, Mass.: Adams Media Corporation, 1996.

PAIN AND INTIMACY

Epps, Roselyn Payne, and Susan Cobb Stewart, eds. *The American Medical Women's Association Guide to Sexuality*. New York: Dell Publishing, 1996.

Monga, Trilok N., guest ed. "Sexuality and Disability." *Physical Medicine and Rehabilitation: State of the Art Reviews* 2 (Philadelphia, Penn., 1995).

Sipski, Marca L., and Graig J. Alexander. *Sexual Function in People with Disability and Chronic Illness: A Health Professional's Guide*. Gaithersburg, Md.: Aspen Publications, 1997.

PAIN IN CHILDREN

McCollum, Audrey T. *The Chronically Ill Child: A Guide for Parents and Professionals*, rev. and enl. ed. New Haven: Yale University Press, 1981.

McCue, Kathleen, with Ron Bonn. *How to Help Children through a Parent's Serious Illness: Supportive, Practical Advice from a Leading Child Care Specialist*. New York: St. Martin's Press, 1994.

Ross, Dorothea M., and Sheila A. Ross. *Childhood Pain: Current Issues, Research, and Management*. Baltimore, Md.: Urban and Schwarzenberg, 1988.

Schechter, Neil L., Charles B. Berde, and Myron Yaster, eds. *Pain in Infants, Children, and Adolescents*, 2nd ed. Philadelphia, Penn.: Lippincott Williams and Wilkins, 2003.

Segal, Julia, and John Simkins. *Helping Children with Ill or Disabled Parents: A Guide for Parents and Professionals*. London: Jessica Kingsley Publishers, 1996.

Travis, Georgia. *Chronic Illness in Children: Its Impact on Child and Family*. Stanford, Calif.: Stanford University Press, 1976.

PAIN AND ADDICTION

Colvin, Rod. *Prescription Drug Addiction: The Hidden Epidemic*. Omaha, Neb.: Addicus Books, 2002.

Mogil, Cindy R. *Swallowing a Bitter Pill: How Prescription and Over-the-Counter Drug Abuse Is Ruining Lives—My Story*. Far Falls, N.J.: New Horizon Press, 2001.

Washton, Arnold, and Donna Boundy. *Willpower's Not Enough: Recovering from Addictions of Every Kind.* New York: HarperPerennial, 1990.

West, James W. *The Betty Ford Center Book of Answers: Help for Those Struggling with Substance Abuse and for the People Who Love Them.* New York: Pocket Books, 1997.

PAIN TREATMENT

Frontera, Walter R., and Julie K. Silver. *Essentials of Physical Medicine and Rehabilitation.* Philadelphia, Penn.: Hanley and Belfus, 2002.

Greene, Walter B., ed. *Essentials of Musculoskeletal Care,* 2nd ed. Rosemont, Ill.: American Academy of Orthopaedic Surgeons, 2001.

Kanner, Ronald. *Pain Management Secrets: Questions You Asked . . . on Rounds, in the Clinic, on Oral Exams.* Philadelphia, Penn.: Hanley and Belfus, 1997.

Lennard, Ted A. *Pain Procedures in Clinical Practice,* 2nd ed. Philadelphia, Penn.: Hanley and Belfus, 2000.

Loeser, John D., ed., Stephen H. Butler, C. Richard Chapman, and Dennis C. Turk, associate eds. *Bonica's Management of Pain,* 3rd ed. Philadelphia, Penn.: Lippincott Williams and Wilkins, 2001.

Starlanyl, Devin, and Mary Ellen Copeland. *Fibromyalgia and Chronic Musculoskeletal Pain: A Survival Manual,* 2nd ed. Oakland, Calif.: New Harbinger Publications, 2001.

Swanson, David W. *Mayo Clinic on Chronic Pain.* Rochester, Minn.: Mayo Foundation, 1999.

Windsor, Robert E., and Dennis M. Lox. *Soft Tissue Injuries: Diagnosis and Treatment.* Philadelphia, Penn.: Hanley and Belfus, 1998.

Notes

1. WHAT IS CHRONIC PAIN?

1. International Association for the Study of Pain, Subcommittee on Taxonomy, Classification of Chronic Pain, "Description of Pain Syndromes and Definitions of Pain Terms," *Pain* (1986), Suppl. 3: S1–S225.

2. David B. Morris, *The Culture of Pain* (Berkeley, Calif.: University of California Press, 1991), p. 63.

3. Ibid., pp. 12–14.

4. Patrick Wall, *Pain: The Science of Suffering* (New York: Columbia University Press, 2000), p. 76.

5. *Comprehensive Accreditation Manual for Hospitals: The Official Handbook* (Chicago: Joint Commission on Accreditation of Healthcare Organizations, 2001).

2. EFFECT ON THE COUPLE

1. T. H. Holmes and R. H. Rahe, "The Social Readjustment Rating Scale," *Journal of Psychosomatic Research*, 11 (2) (1967), pp. 213–218.

2. Maggie Strong, *Mainstay* (New York: Penguin Books Ltd., 1989), p. 5.

3. Gregg Piburn, *Beyond Chaos: One Man's Journey Alongside His Chronically Ill Wife* (Atlanta, Calif.: Arthritis Foundation, 1999), p. 68.

4. Chris McGonigle, *Surviving Your Spouse's Chronic Illness* (New York: Henry Holt and Company, Inc., 1999), p. 83.

3. INTIMACY AND SEXUAL ACTIVITY

1. M. L. Sipski and C. J. Alexander, eds., *Sexual Function in People with Disability and Chronic Illness* (Gaithersburg, Md.: Aspen Publishers, Inc., 1997), p. 11.

4. WORK ISSUES

1. D. M. Spengler et al., "Back Injuries in Industry: A Retrospective Study. I. Overview and Cost Analysis," *Spine* 11 (3) (April 1986), pp. 241–245; S. J. Bigos et al., "II. Injury Factors," pp. 246–251; S. J. Bigos et al., "III. Employee-Related Factors," pp. 252–256.

8. THE EXTENDED FAMILY

1. Cheri Register, *The Chronic Illness Experience* (Center City, Minn.: Hazelden, 1999), p. xxii.

9. EMOTIONAL CHANGES AND DEPRESSION

1. Harold S. Kushner, *How Good Do We Have to Be?: A New Understanding of Guilt and Forgiveness* (Boston, Mass.: Little, Brown and Company, 1997), p. 197.
2. Gerald L. Sittser, *A Grace Disguised: How the Soul Grows through Loss* (Grand Rapids, Mich.: Zondervan Publishing House, 1995), p. 36.

10. MEDICATION DEPENDENCE AND ADDICTION

1. Substance Abuse and Mental Health Services Administration, *Results from the 2002 National Survey on Drug Use and Health: National Findings* (Rockville, Md.: Office of Applied Studies, NHSDA Series H-22, DHHS Publication No. SMA 03–3836, 2003).
2. Rod Colvin, *Prescription Drug Addiction: The Hidden Epidemic* (Omaha, Neb.: Addicus Books, Inc., 2002), p. 69.

12. TRADITIONAL TREATMENT OPTIONS

1. *Chronic Pain in America: Roadblocks to Relief Survey,* conducted for American Pain Society, the American Academy of Pain Medicine, and Janssen Pharmaceutica by Roper Starch Worldwide Inc., 01/1999. See www.ampainsoc.org for more information.

AFTERWORD

1. Virginia Woolf, "On Being Ill," in *The Moment and Other Essays* (New York: Harcourt Bract Jovanovich, 1948), p. 9.
2. Margiad Evans, *A Ray of Darkness* (Dallas: Riverman Press, 1952), p. 11.

Acknowledgments

T H I S book is part of a series geared toward helping people who are sick and their families cope with the consequences of illness. My editor, Ann Downer-Hazell, and her colleagues at Harvard University Press provided me with the wonderful opportunity to write this book. Ann's suggestions have greatly helped to shape this work, and I am grateful to her for her insights.

I consulted several colleagues along the way who were generous with their advice and expertise. Dr. Linda Cozzens is a pediatrician who shared some of her stories with me and offered editorial comments on the chapters that involve children. Gill Kulwant is a pharmacist at Spaulding Rehabilitation Hospital who assisted me with medication-related questions. Lynn Forde, Terry Sutherland, and Dorothy Aiello are physical therapists at my center who reviewed my comments on exercise and modalities in the treatment of pain. Anna Zeliger, my research assistant, helped me track down vital information.

I am also appreciative of the unfailing support that I receive from Dr. Walter Frontera, the chairman of my department at Harvard Medical School. Administrators David Storto, Judith Waterston, and Michael Sullivan have all been incredibly helpful and supportive of my work at Spaulding Rehabilitation Hospital. Diana Barrett is an invaluable mentor and a dear friend. Terry Cucuzza and Terry O'Brien are librarians who always know how to get me the information I need. Finally, the staff at my center, the Spaulding-Framingham Outpatient Center, where we treat many people who are in pain, are extremely professional and empathic individuals. I am fortunate to have the opportunity to work side-by-side with them.

In this book I have used many anecdotes that come from my real experiences as a physician who treats people in pain. However, I have changed the names and identifying characteristics of the patients so that they will not be recognizable to themselves or to others. My patients have taught me more about treating chronic pain and how it affects their loved ones than anything I ever learned in medical school. Although there is certainly core information that any doctor needs to learn in a formal classroom setting, the education that I have received from my patients is invaluable. I am grateful to them for helping me become a better doctor.

Index

Abdominal pain, 18
Acute pain, 8, 9–11
Addiction, 109–111
  prevention of, 112–115
  treatment of, 115–117
Adolescents, 69–70
  pain in, 80–82
Alcohol, 38
Alternative medicine practitioner, 121–122
Americans with Disabilities Act, 52–53
Amphetamines, 37
Anger, 28–29, 41
Antianxiety drugs, 38
Anticholinergic drugs, 37
Anticonvulsants, 37
Antidepressants, 37, 38, 39
Antihypertensives, 37
Anti-inflammatory medications. See Non-steroidal anti-inflammatory drugs (NSAIDs)
Antiparkinsonian drugs, 37
Antipsychotics, 37
Anxiety
  medications for, 38
  symptoms of, 102
Appetite, in children, 72
Arthritis, 11, 14

Back pain, 15
  during pregnancy, 61–62
  work-related, 47–48, 50–51
Barbiturates, 37
Behavior
  in children, 71
  pain, 4–5, 6–7

Botulinum toxin injection, 128–129, 130
Breastfeeding, 62
Burney, Fanny, 4

Capsaicin, 128
Carpal tunnel syndrome, 143
Childbearing, 40–41, 57–63
  genetic factors and, 58–59
  planning for, 59–61
Children
  adolescents, 69–70, 80–82
  appetite changes in, 72
  behavior change in, 71
  chronic pain in, 75–85
    adolescents, 80–82
    causes of, 76–78
    control and, 84–85
    honest communication about, 84–85
    parental pressures and, 77–78, 83
    parental response to, 75–76, 82–84
    school-age children, 79–80
    treatment of, 136–137
    very young children, 78–79
  complementary and alternative medicine for, 144–145
  depression in, 71
  dishonest communication with, 66
  effective communication with, 66–67, 68, 74
  mood changes in, 70–71
  parental pain effects on, 64–74
  school-age, 68–69, 79–80
  school performance by, 72–73
  sleep problems in, 71
  suicide risk in, 73–74
  very young, 67–68, 78–79

Chronic pain, 8, 11–14
  diagnosis of, 118–123
  disease-specific, 14–19
  family experience of, 2, 13–14 (see also
    Children; Marriage)
  language of, 4–7
  treatment of (see Pain treatment)
Communication, parent-child, 66–67, 68,
  74
Complementary and alternative medi-
    cine, 139–147
  in children, 144–145
  in chronic pain, 143–144
  controversy over, 142
  family and, 146
  in older individuals, 145–146
  practitioners of, 146–147
Congenital insensitivity to pain, 8
Contraception, 60
Controlled substances, 104–106. See also
    Opioid analgesics
Corticosteroid injection, 128, 130
Couples, 20–34. See also Marriage
Culture, 5–6

Depression, 95–101
  in adolescents, 81
  biological factors in, 96–97
  in children, 71
  family support in, 102–103
  psychological factors in, 97–99
  social factors in, 99
  symptoms of, 101
  treatment of, 99–102
Disability, 52–54
  psychological effects of, 54–55
Diuretics, 38
Divorce, 31–32
Drug abuse, 111–112

Emotional problems, 27–30
  in children, 70–71
  in sexual relationships, 39–41
Employment. See Work-related injury
Endometriosis, 19

Face pain, 15–16
Family. See also Marriage
  extended, 86–94

  helpful reactions of, 90–91
  negative reactions of, 87–90
  patient expectations of, 91–94
  in pain diagnosis, 123
  pain experience of, 2, 13–14
  work-related injury and, 55–56
Fear, 30
Fecundity, 59
Fertility, 59
Fibromyalgia, 12, 17–18
Fight or flight response, 9
Financial status, changes in, 26–27
Foot pain, 19

Gender, 5
Genetic factors, 58–59
Geriatric patient
  complementary and alternative medi-
    cine in, 145–146
  pain treatment in, 137–138
Gibson, Edward H., 8
Grief, 28
Growing pains, 80
Guilt, 30

Headache, 16–17
Heredity, 58–59
Histamine H-2 blockers, 37
Holmes-Rahe Social Readjustment
    Scale, 22, 23–24
Hospitalization, 9–10

Infidelity, 30–32

Kübler-Ross, Elisabeth, 28

Labor, 62
Lifestyle changes
  in pain treatment, 133
  pain-related, 12–14
Litigation
  family stress with, 55–56
  in work-related injury, 49–52

Magical thinking, 67
Marriage, 20–34
  crises in, 30–32
  emotional problems in, 27–30
  financial status loss in, 26–27

healing changes in, 32–34
intimacy loss in, 25–26, 30–32. *See also*
    Sexual relationship
parenting changes in, 24–25
relationship loss in, 21–25
role changes in, 21–25, 31
sexual relationship in, 35–44. *See also*
    Sexual relationship
stressful events in, 22, 23–24
workload changes in, 24–25
Medications
    for pain treatment, 127–129
    sexual dysfunction and, 36–38, 39
Migraine headache, 17
Motor vehicle accident, 46–47
Muscle relaxants, 37
Myofascial pain syndrome, 12, 18

Narcotics. *See* Opioid analgesics
Neck pain, 18
Non-steroidal anti-inflammatory drugs
    (NSAIDs),
    fetal effects of, 60–61
    in treatment, 127–129

Occupation. *See* Work-related injury
Opioid analgesics, 38, 104–106
    abuse of, 111–112
    addiction to, 109–111, 112–115
    physical dependence on, 107–109
    prescription for, 114–115
    tolerance to, 106–107
    withdrawal from, 107
Oral contraceptives, 60

Pain. *See also* Chronic pain
    classification of, 8–14
    definition of, 1
    historical perspective on, 2–4
    insensitivity to, 8
Pain behaviors, 4–5
    elimination of, 6–7
Pain clinic, 122–123, 135
Pain treatment, 124–138. *See also* Com-
    plementary and alternative medi-
    cine
    in children, 136–137
    cold packs for, 131
    equipment for, 132–133

exercise for, 129–131
goals of, 125–126
in hospital, 10
ice massage for, 131
injections for, 128–129, 130
lifestyle changes for, 133
manual therapy for, 132
medications for, 127–129
nonpharmacologic, 126
in older individuals, 137–138
pain clinics for, 135
psychological intervention for, 134
surgery for, 134–135
transcutaneous electrical nerve stimu-
    lation for, 131
Parent(s)
changed behavior in, 24–25
children's communication with, 66–
    67, 68, 74
children's pain and, 75–76, 77–78, 82–
    84
pain in, children's response to, 64–74
Parent-child communication, 66–67, 68,
    74
Peer pressure, in adolescents, 81–82
Pelvic pain, 19
Pregnancy, 61–63
    planning for, 59–61
Primary care doctor, 120–121

Reproduction, 59–61

School performance, 72–73
Sciatica, 15
Sexual abuse, 41
Sexual relationship, 35–44
    emotional problems and, 39–41
    improvement in, 42–44
    loss of, 25–26, 30–32
    medication effects on, 36–38, 39
    physical illness and, 42–44
    physical problems and, 36–39
Sleep problems, in children, 71
Socioeconomic status, 5, 7, 26–27
Specialist doctor, 120–121
Spinal injection, 129, 130
Stressful events, 22, 23–24
Suffering, 12
Suicide risk, in children, 73–74

166   INDEX

Surgery, pain after, 9–10
Surveillance, litigation and, 51

Temporomandibular joint disorders,
    15–16
TENS (transcutaneous electrical nerve
    stimulation), 131
Tension-type headache, 16–17
Trepanning, 3
Trigeminal neuralgia, 16
Trigger-point injection, 128, 130

Unemployment, 52–55. *See also* Work-
    related injury

Virtuous pain, 7–8
Vocational retraining, 53–54

Well Spouse Foundation, 22
Work-related injury
    compensable vs. noncompensable,
        46–47
    disability and, 52–54
    family stress with, 55–56
    litigation on, 49–52
    psychological effects of, 54–55
    return to work after, 48–49, 52
    risk for, 47–48